PREDICTORS OF TREATMENT RESPONSE IN MOOD DISORDERS

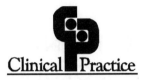

Clinical Practice

Number 34

Judith H. Gold, M.D., F.R.C.P.C.
Elissa P. Benedek, M.D.
Series Editor

PREDICTORS OF TREATMENT RESPONSE IN MOOD DISORDERS

Edited by

Paul J. Goodnick, M.D.

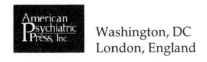

Washington, DC
London, England

Note: The authors have worked to ensure that all information in this book concerning drug dosages, schedules, and routes of administration is accurate as of the time of publication and consistent with standards set by the U.S. Food and Drug Administration and the general medical community. As medical research and practice advance, however, therapeutic standards may change. For this reason and because human and mechanical errors sometimes occur, we recommend that readers follow the advice of a physician who is directly involved in their care or the care of a member of their family.

Copyright © 1996 American Psychiatric Press, Inc.
ALL RIGHTS RESERVED
Manufactured in the United States of America on acid-free paper
First Edition   99   98   97   96   4   3   2   1

American Psychiatric Press, Inc.
1400 K Street, N.W., Washington, DC 20005

Library of Congress Cataloging-in-Publication Data
Predictors of treatment response in mood disorders / Paul J. Goodnick.
    p.   cm. — (Clinical practice ; no. 34)
   Includes bibliographical references and index.
   ISBN 0-88048-494-2
   1. Affective disorders—Chemotherapy.   2. Psychiatry—Differential
therapeutics.   3. Antidepressants—Effectiveness.   4. Psychotropic
drugs—Effectiveness.   5. Electroconvulsive therapy—Evaluation
I. Goodnick, Paul J., 1950–   .   II. Series: Clinical practice ; no.   34
   [DNLM: 1. Treatment Outcome.   2. Antidepressant Agents—
therapeutic use.   3. Antipsychotic Agents—therapeutic use.
4. Affective Disorders—drug therapy.   5. Affective Disorders,
Psychotic—drug therapy.   W1 CL767J no. 34 1994 / QV 77.5 P923 1994]
RC537.P6925   1994
616.85'27061—dc20
DNLM/DLC
for Library of Congress   95-15494
                                                                            CIP

British Library Cataloguing in Publication Data
A CIP record is available from the British Library.

This book is dedicated to my patients, my teachers, and my parents, but especially to my wife and children, who have sacrificed from their time with me; and the Almighty, who has given me the health and opportunity to complete this work.

Contents

Contributors

John Aliapoulous, M.D.
Resident in Psychiatry, University of California at San Diego, San Diego, California

Charles L. Bowden, M.D.
Professor and Director of Biological Psychiatry, University of Texas at San Antonio, San Antonio, Texas

David L. Dunner, M.D.
Professor and Vice Chairman of Psychiatry, University of Washington, Seattle, Washington

S. Hossein Fatemi, M.D., Ph.D.
Resident, Laboratory of Biological Psychiatry, Case Western Reserve University School of Medicine, Cleveland, Ohio

Paul J. Goodnick, M.D.
Professor and Director, Mood Disorders Program, Department of Psychiatry, University of Miami School of Medicine, Miami, Florida

James W. Jefferson, M.D.
Distinguished Senior Scientist, Dean Foundation, and Clinical Professor of Psychiatry, University of Wisconsin, Madison, Wisconsin

Paul E. Keck, Jr., M.D.
Associate Professor of Psychiatry, University of Cincinnati, Cincinnati, Ohio

Susan L. McElroy, M.D.
Associate Professor of Psychiatry, University of Cincinnati, Cincinnati, Ohio

Herbert Y. Meltzer, M.D.
Douglas G. Bond Professor and Director of Biological
Psychiatry, Case Western Reserve University, School of
Medicine, Cleveland, Ohio

Mitchell S. Nobler, M.D.
Fellow in Biological Psychiatry, New York State Psychiatric
Institute and Columbia University, New York, New York

Raymond Ownby, M.D.
Resident in Psychiatry, University of Miami School of
Medicine, Miami, Florida

Harold A. Sackeim, Ph.D.
Professor and Director of Biological Psychiatry, New York State
Psychiatric Institute and Columbia University, New York,
New York

Scott A. West, M.D.
Fellow in Biological Psychiatry, University of Cincinnati,
Cincinnati, Ohio

Sidney Zisook, M.D.
Professor and Director of Research and Training, Department
of Psychiatry, University of California at San Diego, San Diego,
California

Introduction
to the Clinical Practice Series

*O*ver the years of its existence, the series of monographs entitled *Clinical Insights* gradually became focused on providing current, factual, and theoretical material of interest to the clinician working outside of a hospital setting. To reflect this orientation, the name of the Series has been changed to *Clinical Practice.*

The Clinical Practice Series will provide books that give the mental health clinician a practical, clinical approach to a variety of psychiatric problems. These books will provide up-to-date literature reviews and emphasize the most recent treatment methods. Thus, the publications in the Series will interest clinicians working both in psychiatry and in the other mental health professions.

Each year a number of books will be published dealing with all aspects of clinical practice. In addition, from time to time when appropriate, the publications may be revised and updated. Thus, the Series will provide quick access to relevant and important areas of psychiatric practice. Some books in the Series will be authored by a person considered to be an expert in that particular area; others will be edited by such an expert, who will also draw together other knowledgeable authors to produce a comprehensive overview of that topic.

Some of the books in the Clinical Practice Series will have their foundation in presentations at an annual meeting of the American Psychiatric Association. All will contain the most recently available information on the subjects discussed. Theoretical and scientific data will be applied to clinical situations, and case illustrations will be utilized in order to make the material even more relevant for the practitioner. Thus, the Clinical Practice Series should provide educational reading in a compact format especially designed for the mental health clinician–psychiatrist.

Judith H. Gold, M.D., F.R.C.P.C.
Series Editor
Clinical Practice Series

Clinical Practice Series Titles

The Neuroleptic Malignant Syndrome and Related Conditions (#6)
By Arthur Lazarus, M.D., Stephan C. Mann, M.D., and Stanley N. Caroff, M.D.

Anxiety: New Findings for the Clinician (#5)
Edited by Peter Roy-Byrne, M.D.

Anxiety and Depressive Disorders in the Medical Patient (#4)
By Leonard R. Derogatis, Ph.D., and Thomas N. Wise, M.D.

Family Violence: Emerging Issues of a National Crisis (#3)
Edited by Leah J. Dickstein, M.D., and Carol C. Nadelson, M.D.

Divorce as a Developmental Process (#2)
Edited by Judith H. Gold, M.D., F.R.C.P.C.

Treating Chronically Mentally Ill Women (#1)
Edited by Leona L. Bachrach, Ph.D., and Carol C. Nadelson, M.D.

Introduction

*R*ecently, it has been estimated that the cost of depression in the United States in 1990 reached a high of approximately $43.7 billion (Greenberg et al. 1993). Of this amount, $12.4 billion (28%) went toward the direct costs of inpatient hospitalization, outpatient visits, and costs of medication; $7.5 billion (17%) was the cost of loss of lifetime earnings due to depression-related suicide; and $23.8 billion (55%) was due to the cost of work absenteeism and reduced productivity.

Thus, as health care costs are increasingly scrutinized, it becomes imperative to maximize the benefit of the money that is spent to control both the direct and indirect costs of depressive illness. The use of antidepressants in the treatment of mood disorders is an example. Despite their overall effectiveness, results recently indicated that among 201 patients with diverse symptoms of depression and anxiety, fewer than 50% showed evidence of full recovery one year after initial evaluation and treatment (Ormel et al. 1993). Such outcome-related research provides important guidelines for the primary practitioner on choosing an initial treatment for a mood disorder that would reduce the severity and duration of its morbidity. As another example, recent results indicated that patients who received prepaid treatment fared worse than those who received fee-for-service treatment (Rogers et al. 1993). The authors of that paper suggested that "lower treatment levels" of antidepressant medications may have been a reason for the worse outcome.

Consequently, it makes sense, both scientifically and economically, to examine our current state of knowledge on the prediction of response in mood disorders, specifically depression and manic depression. Mania, for example, with a primary indication for lithium treatment, has been associated with lithium "resistance" at a rate of up to 30% of patients (Goodwin and Jamison 1990). In this context, the first three chapters of this book discuss antidepressants: the tricyclic antidepressants, the monoamine oxidase inhibitors, and the newer antidepressants (mostly SSRIs). The next four chapters address treatments for mania: lithium, carbamazepine, valproate, and neuroleptics. The remaining treatment chapter examines electroconvulsive therapy. The final chapter of the book consists of a review and a look forward to future treatment issues.

Chapter 1 by Drs. Aliapoulous and Zisook looks at the tricyclic antidepressants (TCAs) and discusses what has been learned about them since imipramine's introduction in 1954. From that one parent drug, six new TCAs followed within the next decade. The most recent introduction of a TCA in the United States was clomipramine, released by the FDA around 1990. Evidence is reviewed on factors that affect the clinical utility of TCAs: age, personality, family history, and the onset, course, severity, and subtypes of depression. Possible and probable biological predictors of response to TCAs—including acute reaction to psychostimulants, the monamine metabolite "story," and neuroendocrine challenges—are then examined.

In Chapter 2, Dr. Ownby and I look at the parameters of predicting response to the monoamine oxidase inhibitors (MAOIs). An attempt is made to critically review the specific usefulness of MAOIs in atypical (hypersomnic/hyperphagic) depression, as well as the status of baseline platelet MAO, and to determine the strength of the evidence that increased platelet MAO leads to better response. Also, a brief discussion is offered regarding moclobemide, the reversible MAO (RIMA) which is already available in Canada and may soon be distributed in the United States. The treatment profile of this unique medication is compared and contrasted to the profiles of previous MAOIs. Moclobemide appears to be more effective for those depressions in which general MAOIs are less successful (i.e., melancholia), but less effective in atypical depression where general MAOIs may be the treatment of choice.

In Chapter 3, the discussion on newer antidepressants first focuses on the biochemical and clinical parameters that may correlate with response to selective serotonin uptake inhibitors (SSRIs) and bupropion. SSRIs have rapidly become the first-line treatment for major depression. The first SSRI was fluoxetine, which quickly garnered the largest share of the antidepressant medication market upon its release in the United States in January 1988; sertraline (released in February 1992) and paroxetine (released in February 1993) are new additions to this group of medications. Other SSRIs, including fluvoxamine, which is currently prescribed in Canada, may soon become available in the United States. Because SSRIs cost more than TCAs, it is important to be able to predict as closely as possible the response to SSRIs both as a group and individually, whether patients require more serotonin-specific (sertraline, paroxetine) or less serotonin-specific (fluoxetine, fluvoxamine) drugs. The relative current and potential value of baseline serotonin assessments is reviewed as possible fertile ground for widespread clinical application. Clinically, the discussion focuses on symptoms (e.g., psychomotor retardation and fluoxetine response), subtypes of depression (e.g., atypical and bipolar depression), and associated disorders (e.g., obsessive-compulsive disorder). Some evidence exists that might lead a practitioner to choose among the five newer antidepressants according to a particular set of symptoms, and perhaps expect an earlier and better response.

Chapters 4–7 examine medications used in the treatment of mania. In Chapter 4, Dr. Jefferson looks at the positive (e.g., classic history of bipolar disorder) and the purported negative (dysthymic mania and rapid-cycling) predictors of response to lithium. Also, a critical review of the available information on the biological prediction of lithium response is offered.

Due to both the lack of response to lithium and its multiple side effects, patient compliance to a lithium regimen is often quite low. Subsequently, the use of carbamazepine and valproate, both more costly than lithium, has become widespread. Questions regarding whether they are overused, whether they have a predictable response rate at least as good as lithium when used as first-line treatment, and when they should be used instead of lithium are critically addressed by Dr. Bowden in Chapter 5 (on carbamazepine) and Drs. West, McElroy, and Keck, Jr in Chapter 6 (on valproate). Chapter 5 also includes a review of clinical predictors to carbamazepine that are often widely accepted without critique: bipolar depression, mixed mania, rapid-cycling, severity, and family history related to clinical factors. This information is then applied to practical case situations. Dr. West and associates offer a careful separation of predictors of antimanic and antidepressant response to valproate in Chapter 6. Factors that are considered include course of illness, comorbid psychiatric diagnoses, and neurological factors. These help to give the clinician a clear understanding of when to use valproate in the bipolar patient to maximize its usefulness.

In Chapter 7, Drs. Meltzer and Fatemi focus on the long-neglected use of neuroleptics in the treatment of mood disorders and what is known concerning the prediction of response to them. The advent of the atypical neuroleptics, particularly clozapine, has led to improvement of both positive and negative "schizophrenic" symptoms. Although perhaps an oversimplification, positive symptoms are seen as related to mania, whereas negative symptoms are seen as related to depression. Despite the high cost of these newer neuroleptics, their dual dopamine/serotonin activity and a decreased risk of induction of extrapyramidal symptoms and tardive dyskinesia make them potentially good alternative medications.

Having covered the most frequent first-line treatments for both depression and mania, the remaining area to be addressed is electroconvulsive therapy (ECT). This somatic treatment has been used longer than any other, but in terms of when it should or should not be used as a treatment for mania and depression, it is perhaps the least understood. In Chapter 8, Drs. Nobler and Sackeim review the data for the use of ECT in subtypes of depression (e.g., delusional depression), as well as factors such as past treatment history. Critical comment on the usefulness of biological tests like the dexamethasone suppression test is offered. A particular focus of importance for clinicians is the review of items in this chapter that are part of the ECT process and yet predict the response to it (e.g., cerebral blood flow).

Finally, in Chapter 9, Dr. Dunner provides an overview of the predictability of response to somatic treatments in mood disorders. On a conservative basis, the current accepted state of knowledge on predictors is reviewed, while certain myths regarding predictability that have not held up over time are debunked. After the previous authors' presentations of those factors that appear to be predictors (and which may hold up in the future), a sobering insight is offered regarding the relative lack of established predictors in a society so conscious of health-care costs.

It is hoped and expected that upon completion of this volume, the reader will identify the following for each patient presenting with a mood disorder: 1) the key questions to ask and symptoms to assess during the initial meeting (regarding both depression/mania and other psychiatric syndromes); 2) the clinical laboratory tests that may be useful to obtain; 3) the *research* laboratory techniques that may be of use; and 4) the occasions when a psychological profile would be helpful. It is anticipated that with this guidance, the general clinician will be able to treat patients more quickly and successfully.

References

Goodwin FK, Jamison KR: Manic-Depressive Illness. New York & Oxford, Oxford University Press, 1990

Greenberg PE, Stiglin LE, Finkelstein SN, et al: The economic burden of depression in 1990. J Clin Psychiatry 54:405–418, 1993.

Ormel J, Oldehinkel T, Brilman E, et al: Outcome of depression and anxiety in primary care. Arch Gen Psychiatry 50:759–766, 1993

Rogers WH, Wells KB, Meredith LS, et al: Outcomes for adult outpatients with depression under prepaid or fee-for-service financing. Arch Gen Psychiatry 50:517–525, 1993

Acknowledgments

I would like to thank Teresa Van Norman and her associates, Cheryl Clemence and Faith Martin, at the University of Miami Department of Psychiatry, for their assistance in editing and preparing this manuscript. My thanks to Cecilia Jorge, M.D., for reviewing the galleys. I would also like to extend my appreciation to Dr. Judith Gold, Claire Reinburg, and Pamela Harley at APPI for their helpful suggestions.

CHAPTER 1

Tricyclic Antidepressant Medications

John Aliapoulous, M.D., and Sidney Zisook, M.D.

Since their introduction for the treatment of depression in the 1950s, tricyclic antidepressants (TCAs) have enhanced the quality of life for millions of individuals with major mood disorders. Indeed, the development of TCAs may be the major contribution psychiatry has made to the field of medicine in the last three to four decades. Unfortunately, however, this class of medications is far from perfect, and perhaps 20%–30% of individuals with disabling major depression do not respond fully to TCAs, whereas many others respond only partially or are unable to tolerate therapeutic doses because of side effects. In some cases, side effects are only nuisances; but in others, side effects are serious and may prevent individuals from taking adequate doses of their antidepressant medications, impede compliance, or lead to serious or even fatal complications, especially when used by medically ill patients, or the elderly, or when individuals overdose with TCAs. Thus, it is always important to assess the risk-benefit ratio before prescribing TCAs, and to know which depressed patients are most likely to benefit from a particular antidepressant medication.

The need for clinicians to be able to predict which depressed patients will respond to TCAs is buttressed by the availability of alternate therapies for the treatment of major depression. Thus, several studies have attempted to identify predictors of response to TCAs. Unfortunately, the results of these studies have not yet lead to a consensus. There are several reasons for this failure, including 1) the heterogeneity of depression (Akiskal 1989; Brockington et al. 1982; Caine et al. 1994; Farmer and McGuffin 1989; Kendall 1976; Zimmerman et al. 1986), 2) diagnostic imprecision and different diagnostic criteria or nosological conventions used in various studies, 3) variability in the course of mood disorders, 4) comorbidity (which is often ignored in these trials), 5) the fact that not all TCAs are alike (Richelson 1991), and 6) the usual methodological problems seen in clinical trials such as small samples of patients with diverse disorders, lack of standardization of outcome measures, and inadequate comparison of control groups. In addition, many of the studies on patients who do not respond to TCAs included heterogeneous groups of depressed patients who were treated for short periods of time with doses of TCAs that are now considered subtherapeutic (Roose et al. 1986). Studying a large number of patients who had been labeled as having "treatment-refractory depression," Schatzberg and colleagues (1983) reported that only 30% of the patients had received what these researchers considered to be adequate tricyclic treatment. Perhaps the greatest predictors of a poor response to TCAs are an inadequate dose or duration of treatment (Lydiard 1985).

Despite the above methodological problems and other sources of variances in studies looking at predictors of response, and the lack of consistent or conclusive findings, two excellent clinical review articles include evaluations of predictive studies completed up to the point of their publications. In the first of these, Bielski and Friedel (1976) critically reviewed all prospective double-blind studies on imipramine and amitriptyline published up to the mid-1970s. Their review pointed out that most demographic, personality, past history, family history, course of illness, symptom, and biochemical predictors had not been consistently validated. On the other hand, Bielski and Friedel's review found relatively consistent evidence that upper socioeconomic class, insidious onset, anorexia, weight loss, middle and late insomnia, and psychomotor retardation predict response to TCAs. The predictors of a poor response (i.e., where TCAs are no better than the placebo treatment) were neurotic, hypochondriacal, and hysterical traits, multiple prior episodes, and delusions. Bielski and Friedel reviewed some preliminary data suggesting low pretreatment levels of urinary 3-methoxy-4-hydroxyphenylglycol

(MHPG) may predict response to imipramine, whereas high levels of MHPG may predict response to amitriptyline, but they cautioned that more work needs to be done on these potential biological predictors.

In the second of these comprehensive reviews, Joyce and Paykel (1989) concluded that depressed patients with a good premorbid personality, an insidious onset of depression, psychomotor retardation, and an intermediate level of severity and "endogenicity," but without psychotic features, may be the patients who respond best to TCAs. Although Joyce and Paykel felt biological predictors of response to TCAs may be important in the long run, their routine clinical usefulness was not yet sufficiently established—a conclusion not unlike that voiced by Bielski and Friedel some 13 years earlier.

Both of the reviews previously described predated the widespread use of the selective serotonin reuptake inhibitors (SSRIs) and bupropion. In addition, other novel, non-TCA antidepressants are soon to be introduced and will broaden clinicians' armamentarium against depression, while simultaneously increasing their choices. Like the TCAs before them, these newer medications do not work for all depressed patients and are associated with their own unique side effect profiles (Feighner and Boyer 1991; Zisook and Andia 1992). Thus, more than ever, it is important to be able to predict which class of medications, or specific medication within that class, is likely to be the most effective—and safest—for each depressed person.

In this chapter we review information on predictors of response to TCAs. A special emphasis will be given to studies that were completed since publication of the aforementioned reviews. Although investigators and clinicians alike are increasingly cognizant of the chronic and highly recurrent nature of depressive disorders and also of the need to consider both maintenance and long-term prevention in the treatment plans for depressed individuals (Keller et al. 1992; Kupfer et al. 1992; Wells et al. 1992), in this chapter we will emphasize the predictors of response to acute treatment (response and remission) rather than concentrate on maintenance phases (Frank et al. 1991). A brief review of the personal and family history predictors is followed by a discussion of the social and clinical predictors and a review of biological predictors.

Personal and Familial Predictors

Demography

Sex.   There is no convincing evidence from controlled studies that sex is a predictor of response to TCAs.

Age.   Of the earlier studies reviewed by Bielski and Friedel (1976) that looked at demographic factors (Abraham et al. 1963; Deykin and DiMascio 1972; Rickels et al. 1964), most failed to show the predictive ability of the variable age; however, a series of studies from the National Institute of Mental Health (NIMH) Collaborative Depression Study Group (Raskin 1974) demonstrated the efficacy of imipramine compared with chlorpromazine or placebo only in depressed patients over the age of 40. Similarly, Kiloh and colleagues (1962) found that an age of 40 or older predicted a good response to imipramine in depressed outpatients. In contrast, however, in an inpatient study of depressed women, older patients were poor responders to imipramine (Wittenborn et al. 1973). More recently, some studies showing that older age predicts a poor response to TCAs (Brown and Brawley 1983; Sotsky et al. 1991) contradict others studies (Sorensen et al. 1978). Despite the lack of a consensus regarding age as a predictor of response, several studies have documented that older persons with major depression often benefit from TCAs (Gerson et al. 1988; Jenike 1989; Salzman 1994). In one study on TCA treatment of late-life depression, Georgotas and colleagues (1989) found that lower plasma levels of nortriptyline in the early weeks of treatment were associated with a longer time to response. In another study, Katz and colleagues (1990) found nortriptyline effective even for frail older persons with major depression living in an institutional setting. In the later study, patients with the greatest self-care deficits and the lowest levels of serum albumin were the least likely to respond to nortriptyline.

Personality.   Several studies have found that personality traits and disorders influence treatment (Akiskal et al. 1983; Reich and Vasile 1993). For example, there appears to be a consensus that patients with neurotic, hypochondriacal or histrionic personality traits do not respond as well to TCAs as more stable personality types (Bielski and Friedel 1976; Deykin and DiMascio 1972; Downing and Rickels 1973; Hirschfeld et al. 1986; Kiloh et al. 1962; Paykel et al. 1973; Raskin et al. 1970; Shawcross and Tyrer 1985; Weissman et al. 1978). Joffe and Regan (1989) found that certain personality traits (assertiveness, independence, and competitiveness) were associated with a positive response to TCAs, but the presence or absence of a personality disorder per se was not related to outcome. In partial conflict with Joffe and Regan's findings, several studies have concluded that depressed patients with an associated personality disorder do not respond to TCAs as well as patients without personality disorders (Black et al. 1988; Charney and Nelson 1981; Frank et al. 1987; Pfohl et al. 1984; Pilkonis and Frank 1988; Thompson et al. 1988). In the NIMH Treatment of Depression Collaborative Research Program, depressed patients with personality disorders had a significantly worse outcome in social functioning than patients without personality disorders and were more likely to have residual symptoms of depression after 16 weeks of treatment. Outcome was similar for patients in each of the three different clusters of personality disorders (i.e., odd-eccentric, dramatic-erratic and anxious-fearful). Contrary to initial expectations, depressed patients with personality disorders did not do better in psychotherapeutic treatment than in pharmacotherapy with TCAs (Shea et al. 1990).

Finally, one study that did not find that personality disorders predict poor response to antidepressant treatment bears mention. In that outpatient chart review study, Downs and colleagues (1992) reported that although depressed patients with concomitant personality disorder initially were more functionally impaired than patients with major depression alone, they actually improved as much as patients with major depression alone; patients with concomitant borderline personality disorder showed the most impairment before treatment, as well as the most improvement with treatment. A medication clinic was the predominant treatment setting for patients from both groups, and antidepressants, primarily TCAs, were the most frequently prescribed class of medications. Patients with concomitant personality disorders, however, were more likely to receive a polypharmacy of TCAs plus antipsychotics or benzodiazepines. This finding supports the possibility that although previous studies may be correct in their finding that concomitant personality disorders predict a poor response in depressed patients who are treated with TCAs alone, this refractory tendency may be overcome by aggressive augmentation with other medications. Clearly, this hypothesis requires testing with controlled, prospective trials.

Personal or family history. Although the data are relatively sparse, most clinicians feel that a history of response to TCAs, or to a specific TCA, during a previous episode of major depression predicts a response to the same medication during the current episode (Angst 1961; Pare and Mack 1971); however, there are exceptions to this general rule (Fakhr El-Islam 1973), as well as some evidence that the likelihood of recovery with TCAs may decrease with each subsequent episode (Cassano et al. 1983; Keller et al. 1986b; Roose et al. 1986).

Some investigators have suggested that the tendency to respond to a specific class of antidepressant medication runs in families (Pare et al. 1971). Other family history predictors are sparse and generally have not been replicated. Raskin and colleagues (1970) observed that patients who respond to imipramine were more likely to have mothers with histories of psychiatric disturbances than patients who do not respond; Deykin and Dimascio (1972) reported that depressed patients with histories of maternal death before age 15 and of paternal psychiatric difficulties responded poorly to amitriptyline; and Akiskal (1982) found that incomplete recovery in patients with primary depressive illness treated with TCAs was associated with a positive family history of affective disorders.

> *Case 1.*   The patient is a 22-year-old woman whose mother and older sister had both previously responded quickly and completely to amitriptyline. When she presented for psychiatric treatment of her severe major depression, she also complained of weight gain, low energy, and constipation. Therefore, to avoid antihistaminic and anticholinergic side effects, she was prescribed 20 mg of fluoxetine daily rather than amitriptyline. Because of minimal therapeutic response by the 4th week of treatment, her daily dose was increased to 40 mg, then to 60 mg daily after the 6th week. Although she noted some improvement in mood, outlook, and overeating, she re-

mained mildly to moderately depressed after 8 weeks of treatment. Because of the inadequate response, and on the basis of her family history, fluoxetine was discontinued and amitriptyline begun, initially in doses of 75 mg each night, but increasing to 150 mg nightly by the 10th day of treatment. Within 2 weeks, she was feeling "back to normal." Her weight had stabilized, energy improved, and she had minimal side effects. Her excellent clinical response continued over the next several months of treatment.

Social and Clinical Predictors

Life Events

It has long been felt that life events are related to the onset of depressive episodes (Brown et al. 1973; Paykel et al. 1969), but less is known about the role of life events as modulators of response. In a study of 80 outpatients with nonbipolar primary depressions, Lloyd and colleagues (1981) found that events occurring in the year before beginning treatment (antecedent events) with TCAs were unrelated to medication response. Their findings have been replicated in other studies (Garvey et al. 1984; Hirschfeld et al. 1986). What was unique about Lloyd and colleagues' study was that they also looked at events occurring during the treatment period itself (concurrent events), and found that these events were related to outcome. In particular, a poor TCA response was associated with events that were undesirable, health related, and perceived as being outside the patient's own control. Similarly, Akiskal (1982) has reported that a poor response to full doses of two to three TCAs given in therapeutic trials of 2 months each was significantly correlated with concurrent, incapacitating medical diseases (including the use of depressant antihypertensives), multiple object loss through death of immediate family members, and having a disabled spouse.

Patient Expectations

There is surprisingly little literature on the relationship of patient expectations of outcome with actual improvement. In the NIMH Treatment of Depression Collaborative Research Program, patients who had low expectations for improvement with treatment did not responded to imipramine as well as patients with high expectations (Sotsky et al. 1991). Thus, positive expectations and hope may predict improvement.

Onset and Course of Depression

An insidious onset of depression has been found to predict a good response to imipramine (Kiloh et al. 1962; Raskin et al. 1970). Several studies also have suggested that depressions of shorter duration show more likelihood of improving than more chronic depressions (Bielski and Friedel 1976; Keller et al. 1992; Rush et al. 1983), but there is still some controversy about the relationship between duration of depression and response to TCAs (Joyce and Paykel 1989; Kupfer and Spiker 1981; Loyd and Tsuang 1985). The literature also partially supports the view that more previous episodes of depression predict a poorer response than fewer episodes (Bielski and Friedel 1976; Cassano et al. 1983; Joyce and Paykel 1989); however, in a large multicentered naturalistic study of patients with major depression, many, but not all of whom were treated with TCAs, Keller and colleagues (1986b) reported that although the number of previous episodes of depression predicted recurrence of future depression, it did not predict recovery time for the current episode. Indeed, in a study of treatment of consecutive episodes of major depression in the elderly with nortriptyline and interpersonal psychotherapy, Reynolds and co-workers (1994) found that not only were recurrent episodes of major depression treatable, but also that most patients responded more quickly in the subsequent episodes than in the index episode.

Although there are no data showing that patients with recurrent depressions do better with TCAs than do patients with single episodes, there are excellent data that TCAs are useful for preventive treatment in patients with recurrent unipolar depressions who have recovered from their index episode (Kupfer et al. 1992). Such patients should be treated with the full therapeutic dose of TCA (Frank et al. 1990).

There are limited data on whether depressed patients with a history of mania or hypomania (i.e., Bipolar I or Bipolar II) have a different likelihood of response than patients with pure unipolar depression (Keller et al. 1986a), but the possibility of inducing a manic episode or rapid cycling with the TCA must be considered (Akiskal 1983; Bunney 1977; Wehr and Goodwin 1987). Patients who are rapidly cycling between depression and mania or who are in a mixed mood state are less likely to respond or recover with antidepressant medications than bipolar patients in a more classic, pure depressive state (Keller et al. 1986a). Finally, there is growing evidence that bipolar depressions may not be as responsive to TCAs as they are to MAOIs (Thase et al. 1992; Himmelhoch et al. 1991).

Severity of Depression

In the NIMH Treatment of Depression Collaborative Research Program, which compared psychotherapy, imipramine, and case management for patients with major depression, differences among treatments were present only for the subgroups of patients who were more severely depressed and impaired at baseline. Severity was defined as a pretreatment 17-item Hamilton Depression Rating Scale (HDRS) score of 20 or more and a Global Assessment Scale (GAS) score of 50 or more. Although there was some evidence of the effectiveness of interpersonal therapy with severely depressed patients, there was much stronger evidence of the effectiveness of imipramine in these patients. In contrast, neither case management nor cognitive therapy were very effective for patients with severe depression, and there were no significant differences among any of the treatment conditions for the less severely depressed or functionally impaired patients (Elkin et al. 1989). In a secondary analysis of this data, Sotsky and colleagues (1991) amplified these original findings by showing that not only did patients with the highest depression severity scores respond best to imipramine, but, in particular, work dysfunction was the single most robust predictor of good outcome with imipramine.

It is possible that the rate of response of very severe depressions (mean HDRS score = 33; GAS = 35) to TCAs may be less satisfactory than that of moderate depression (mean HDRS score = 21; GAS = 49), but this is based largely on one inpatient study that used adequate doses of TCAs for only 4 weeks (Kocis et al. 1990). For many patients, 4 weeks may not be a long enough trial. Thus, rather than being less responsive to TCAs than moderately severe depression, "very severe" depression may simply take longer to respond. This area needs further study.

Specific Symptoms of Depression

For the most part, individual symptoms of depression have not been found to be consistent predictors of a good therapeutic response to TCAs (Bielski and Friedel 1976; Joyce and Paykel 1989; Klein and Davis 1980; Stern et al. 1980). As Stern and colleagues (1980) point out, clinical lore suggests that depressed patients who are anxious or have trouble sleeping respond better to sedating TCAs, such as amitriptyline or doxepin, whereas patients with retarded depression do better on more stimulating TCAs, such as protriptyline or desipramine, or, conversely, with SSRIs or bupropion. This speculation, however, has not been empirically validated by controlled studies. The few symptoms reported to predict good response to TCAs in Bielski and Friedel's review (1976) include psychomotor retardation, poor appetite, weight loss, middle insomnia, and early morning awakening; however, there is controversy over the specificity of sleep or appetite disturbances as predictors of response to TCAs (Joyce and Paykel 1989). Comparing depressed outpatients with mood reactivity in a randomized trial comparing imipramine, phenelzine, and placebo, McGrath and colleagues (1992) reported that patients who had either oversleeping, overeating, severe anergia, or pathological rejection sensitivity had an inferior response to imipramine. Finally, Klein (1974) has suggested that pervasive anhedonia (i.e., mood nonreactivity) is the key feature of a TCA-sensitive dysphoria, but this finding has not been consistently replicated. It is interesting that most of the symptoms that have been implicated as predictors of response to TCAs overlap with symptoms often seen in severe depression and in depressions that are considered melancholic or endogenous.

Specific Syndromes and Subtypes of Depression

Melancholia.   Since the introduction of TCAs, researchers have examined the relationship between the melancholic subtype and treatment response. Several (Klein 1974; Paykel 1972; Raskin and

Crook 1976), but not all (Abraham et al. 1963; Simpson et al. 1976) of the earlier studies found that the melancholic subtype—or its forerunner and close relative, endogenous depression—responds better to TCAs than nonmelancholic or nonendogenous depressions. Interpretation of these early studies, however, is hampered by the reliance on unspecified or nonoperational criteria for diagnosing melancholia (Zimmerman and Spitzer 1989).

Because of the potential utility of melancholia as a treatment predictor, the DSM-III introduced the subtype "melancholia" and provided operational criteria (American Psychiatric Association 1980). In the years following the publication of DSM-III, however, several studies called into question whether the DSM-III criteria for melancholia predicted treatment response. Reviewing this issue as part of the American Psychiatric Workgroup to Revise DSM-III, Zimmerman and Spitzer (1989) reviewed 12 treatment studies that concluded that melancholic patients were not more likely to respond to somatic treatment than nonmelancholic patients (Nelson et al. 1990). Many of these studies evaluated response to TCAs and did not find that melancholia predicted response to TCAs (Coryell and Turner 1985; Kupfer and Spiker 1981; Paykel et al. 1982; Prusoff et al. 1980; Rickels et al. 1964; Stewart et al. 1983; Zimmerman et al. 1985).

To provide a new definition of melancholia that might better predict treatment outcome, the criteria for DSM-III-R were changed and included, as one of its nine items, "previous good response to specific and adequate somatic antidepressant treatment" (American Psychiatric Association 1987). Comparing the DSM-III and the DSM-III-R criteria for melancholia in hospitalized depressed patients treated without medications versus patients treated with desipramine, Nelson and colleagues (1990) found the two criteria sets more similar than dissimilar; neither predicted a drug response that distinguished itself from that of nonmelancholics. On the other hand, both criteria sets identified patients who are not likely to respond to hospitalization alone. TCA response was similar in patients with and without melancholia, but only desipramine provided significantly more help than hospitalization alone in patients with melancholia. Thus, it appears that both melancholic and nonmelancholic patients respond to TCAs, but the greatest differences between drug and placebo treatment, and perhaps also between drug and psychotherapy treatment as well (Peselow et al. 1992; Prusoff et al. 1980), are most likely to occur in depressed patients with melancholia.

Depression with atypical features.   Atypical depressive features include mood reactivity, increased appetite and weight, hypersomnia, sensitivity to emotional rejection, and a sense of severe fatigue that creates a sensation of "leaden paralysis" or extreme heaviness of the arms or legs (Leibowitz et al. 1988). In some concepts of atypical depression, other features, such as extreme anxiety, phobic symptoms, or somatization also are considered atypical features (Davidson et al. 1982; Zisook 1985; Zisook et al. 1993). There is overlap between patients with atypical depression and patients with anergic bipolar depression (Thase 1991). Patients with atypical depressions tend to respond positively to monoamine oxidase inhibitors, but respond less well to TCAs than patients with typical forms of major depression (Quitkin et al. 1988, 1991). McGrath and colleagues (1992) have reported that patients with a "mood-reactive" major depression respond better to monoamine oxidase inhibitors than to TCAs if they have any of the following features when compared with those patients with none of the features: oversleeping, overeating, severe anergy, and pathologic rejection sensitivity.

Depression with psychotic features.   Severe major depression that is associated with hallucinations or delusions tends not to respond to TCAs alone (Charney and Nelson 1981; Glassman and Roose 1981; Spiker et al. 1985). Such depressions have been reported to respond better to combinations of antidepressants and neuroleptics together than to either medication alone (Spiker et al. 1985), and Anton and Sexauer (1990) have reported that amoxapine, a TCA with neuroleptic properties, works as well as amitriptyline plus perphenazine. The treatment of choice for depression with psychotic features most likely is electroconvulsive therapy (Kantor and Glassman 1977).

Depression with Panic Disorder

Major depression and panic disorders often coexist. Approximately 20%–30% of patients with major depression also have a panic disorder (Barlow et al. 1986; Breier et al. 1984), and between

20% and 90% of patients who meet the criteria for panic disorders experience an episode of major depression one or more times during their lives (Lydiard 1991). Grunhaus and colleagues (1986, 1988) reported that hospitalized patients with comorbid panic disorder and major depression who were treated with TCAs did less well than similarly treated patients with major depression alone. Similarly, naturalistic follow-up studies suggest that the prognosis for mixed panic disorder and major depression is poorer than for patients with major depression alone (Coryell et al. 1988; Vollrath and Angst 1989). It is possible that monoamine oxidase inhibitors (MAOIs) may be more effective than TCAs in patients with comorbid major depression and panic disorder (Leibowitz et al. 1988; Robinson et al. 1985).

> *Case 2.* The patient is a 56-year-old woman who had periods of free-floating anxiety, separation anxiety, and episodes of low-grade depression during childhood. Her first of several major depressive episodes occurred after a therapeutic abortion at age 15. After a spontaneous abortion at age 22, she experienced her first panic attack, and over the next few months developed a full-blown panic disorder with agoraphobia. Treatment with an MAOI, phenylzine, effectively treated her panic disorder, but left her still moderately depressed. On the other hand, treatment with TCAs brought her depression into partial remission, but left her vulnerable to intermittent panic attacks. She couldn't take MAOIs and TCAs simultaneously because of side effects (nausea, dizziness, headaches, and lethargy). With both MAOIs and TCAs, low-dose benzodiazepines were necessary to reduce residual anxiety. Because of these partial responses to MAOIs and TCAs through the years in this woman with both major depression and panic disorder, further attempts to treat her most recent major depressive episode with either of these types of medication were not entertained. Instead, she was given a serotonin uptake blocker, paroxetine, and had an excellent and lasting antidepressant, antipanic, and antianxiety response.

Patients With Concurrent Medical Disorders

The prevalence of major depression in patients who are medically ill is substantially higher than in the general population (Cassem 1991; Cohen-Cole and Stoudemire 1987; Katon and Sullivan 1991; Wells et al. 1988). Although depressed patients with concurrent medical illness often derive great benefit from psychopharmacologic treatment of their depressive disorder (Katon and Sullivan 1991), concurrent medical illness may adversely affect response to TCAs (Black et al. 1987; Popkin et al. 1985). In one study of the outcome of antidepressant use in medically ill inpatients, Popkin and colleagues (1985) found that 32% of the patients had to be withdrawn from their medications because of side effects, often including delirium. Only 40% of the patients achieved what the investigators felt to be an adequate response to treatment. Similarly, studying factors associated with incomplete recovery in patients with primary depressive illness, Akiskal (1982) reported that serious or incapacitating medical illness superimposed months to years after the onset of depression adversely affected response to TCAs. A related contributing factor to nonresponse that Akiskal found was use of reserpine or alphamethyldopa for treatment of hypertension. Finally, Akiskal reported that secondary alcoholism, or sedative or hypnotic dependence, prevented recovery from acute primary depression. Thus, concurrent medical illness or substance use may predict a less satisfying response to TCAs than in patients who are medically healthy.

Number of predictors.   One recent study (Nelson et al. 1994) found that 15 of 50 (30%) inpatients with major depression failed to respond adequately to a 4-week desipramine trial in which 24-hour plasma concentration was used to rapidly achieve therapeutic desipramine levels. The strongest correlates of poor response were definite personality disorder, prior treatment failure, near delusional status, and age of 35 years or younger; however, no single item predicted poor response very well, because 91% of patients with one or no predictors responded. On the other hand, in patients with two or more predictors, only 25% responded. Thus, the number of predictors may be another important variable to consider when trying to make rational treatment choices.

Time to response to treatment.   Although patients may show improvement by the end of the 1st week (Katz et al. 1987), most may not fully respond for more than 6–8 weeks (Quitkin et al. 1984, 1987; Zisook and Andia 1992), or even longer in the elderly (Georgotas 1989).
    Although some investigators (Quitkin et al. 1987) have suggested that an early (i.e., within 1 week) response to a TCA is not

a true drug response, others (Coryell et al. 1982; Hodern et al. 1963; Jarvik et al. 1982; Nagayama et al. 1991; Zisook et al. 1982) have found that an early positive response to TCAs may predict overall efficacy. For example, Hodern and colleagues (1963) noted that 1) more than half of their depressed female outpatients treated with amitriptyline showed significant improvement after 1 week; 2) early improvement was a useful prognostic indicator; and 3) middle insomnia, anorexia, and loss of interest and capacity to work significantly differentiated patients who responded early from patients who did not respond. Similarly, in an outpatient study of depressed patients treated with either amitriptyline or amoxapine, Zisook and colleagues (1982) found that 30% of patients showed substantial clinical improvement within 1 week. Patients who responded quickly were somewhat less depressed than patients who did not respond quickly at baseline, and they had less emotional withdrawal, hostility, or interpersonal disturbances, and felt more hopeful, useful, and needed before treatment began. The first symptoms to improve, as early as 4 days after treatment was initiated, included insomnia, weight loss, suicidal ideation, and work or interest disturbances. Most important, the patients who responded quickly maintained their advantage throughout the 4-week study in terms of both symptomatic outcome and treatment adherence. A more recent study completed in Japan (Nagayama et al. 1991) confirmed these earlier findings, demonstrating that the most effective predictor of efficacy in depressed inpatients treated with clomipramine was the percentage improvement in the HDRS scores during the 1st week of treatment.

These data suggest the important question of whether early nonresponse or minimal response to TCAs predicts later nonresponse. That is, if a patient shows minimal response to a TCA after the first few weeks of treatment, should treatment be continued through a full course (6–8 weeks)? Some studies have suggested that patients who show minimal improvement to TCAs after the first few weeks tend not to show therapeutic response later in the trial (Coryell et al. 1982), whereas others have found substantial numbers of patients whose therapeutic response begins only after the first several weeks (Georgotas and McCue 1989; Quitkin et al. 1987). Noting a response rate over the first 7 weeks of treatment of approximately 60% for nortriptyline versus a 13% rate for placebo, Georgotas and McCue (1989) found additional benefit from extending the antidepressant trial 2 more weeks, during which time another 15% of patients responded; furthermore, one-third of the subjects who had not responded by week 9 responded when kept on medication for up to 12 weeks. Georgotas and colleagues (1989) found that lower plasma levels of nortriptyline in the early weeks of treatment were associated with a longer time to response. Although the question of how long to treat before augmenting or changing medications still needs to be resolved with well-designed prospective trials, the authors recommend treating at the full dose of a TCA for at least 6–8 weeks before considering a patient nonresponsive.

> *Case 3.*   The patient is a 65-year-old man who had the onset of his first episode of major depression 6 months before seeking treatment. He was given 100 mg nortriptyline daily. After 4 weeks of treatment, he still had no response to medication. Although there were no side effects, orthostatic changes were minimal, and there were no changes on electrocardiogram, a blood level of nortriptyline was drawn. The test revealed levels well within the nortriptyline window, specifically, 125 µg/ml. He refused to consider any augmentation, as he was extremely frightened of polypharmacy. After 6 weeks of treatment, he remained severely depressed, but refused to change medications, as he didn't want to "start all over." On the morning of his 55th day of treatment, he woke up feeling more energetic and hopeful. Over the next few days, the patient's appetite and sleep improved, and for the first time in months, he noted a wish to live. By the 10th week of treatment, he was in full remission, which continued over the next several months. After approximately 10 months of treatment, nortriptyline was gradually discontinued without any return of depressive symptoms.

Dose.   As noted previously, many of the studies on predictors of response to TCAs either failed to specify the dose or used doses now felt to be subtherapeutic for some depressed patients (Bielski and Friedel 1976; Joyce and Paykel 1989). Although we do not yet know how to predict which patients will require lower or higher doses within the dose range recommended for any particular TCA, we do know that some depressed patients may require doses at least as high as 300 mg of imipramine or its equivalent before the patient can be considered nonresponsive (American Psychiatric Association 1993; Keller et al. 1982; Schatzberg 1991). Blood drug levels have been shown to correlate with beneficial and toxic effects for many TCAs, most notably nortriptyline, desipramine and imipramine (American Psychiatric Association Task Force on the Use of Laboratory Tests in Psychiatry 1985). For nortriptyline especially, blood level determination may help maximize response because of wide variation in blood levels achieved between individuals with any given dose and a fairly narrow window of ideal blood levels. Thus, a substantial proportion of patients who do not respond to a dose as low as 150 mg of nortriptyline may respond after a dose reduction to achieve therapeutic blood levels (Kragh-Sorensen et al. 1976).

A summary of the social and clinical factors that may predict a poor response to TCAs is outlined in Table 1–1.

Table 1–1. Summary of "probable" nonbiological predictors of a poor response to TCAs

- Neurotic, hypochondriacal, or histrionic traits
- Concomitant personality disorder
- Past personal nonresponse to a particular agent
- Past nonresponse in first-degree blood relative
- Parents with psychiatric disturbances or mother who died before age 15
- Concomitant negative life events
- Low expectation of improvement
- Long duration of present or most recent episode
- Severe depression
- Overeating, oversleeping, severe anergia, severe sensitivity to rejection
- Delusions or hallucinations
- Comorbid panic disorder
- Concurrent medical disorder
- More than one predictor of poor response
- Lack of early improvement in symptoms
- Inadequate duration or dose of treatment

Biological Predictors

Mood Response to Psychostimulants

An initial report by Fawcett and Sionopolous (1971), in which a positive (mood-brightening) pretreatment response to stimulants was highly correlated with a 4-week response to imipramine or desipramine, was replicated by van Kammen and Murphy (1978) with imipramine, by Spar and La Rue (1985) with desipramine, and by Sabelli and colleagues (1983) with both imipramine and desipramine. At the same time, preliminary data suggested that a dysphoric or neutral response to stimulants may be associated with subsequent therapeutic response to nortriptyline (Sabelli et al. 1983) or amitriptyline (Brown and Brawley 1983; Sabelli et al. 1983); however, neither Ettigi and colleagues (1983) nor Faber and colleagues (1989) were able to replicate Fawcett and Sionopoulos' original finding with regard to desipramine, and at least one study (Quadri et al. 1980) found that patients who respond to mood brighteners improved with amitriptyline. Thus, the initial hope that an amphetamine challenge might help differentiate depressed patients who had a noradrenergic-mediated response to desipramine or imipramine from a more serotonergic-mediated response to amitriptyline were not completely borne out by subsequent studies. These studies validate the heterogeneity of depression, but the potential utility of psychostimulant response to help identify different drug responses to different TCAs has not yet been realized.

Case 4.   The patient is a 31-year-old man who has had a low-grade depression marked by dysphoric mood, low self-esteem, chronic insomnia, and poor concentration for most of his adult life. Over the past 3 months he noted an acute worsening of his mood, along with anhedonia, neurovegetative symptoms, and suicidal ideation in the context of a recent divorce. Although he was not abusing alcohol and other substances at the time, he had a past history of both amphetamine and cocaine abuse. The only time he ever felt energetic or positive about life was when he took psychostimulants. On the basis of his previous mood-brightening response to psychostimulants, he was given a relatively specific norepinephrine uptake blocker, desipramine. After 4 weeks on a daily dose of 200 mg of desipramine, he no longer felt depressed. Not only did symptoms of his major depressive episode remit, but so did symptoms of his underlying dysthymia. The patient has remained on 200 mg of desipramine over the past 3 years. Each attempt to discontinue the desipramine or even decrease the dose has been met with a recurrence of depressive symptoms.

Monoamine metabolites. Despite a multitude of methodologic problems involved in obtaining, measuring, and interpreting catecholamine metabolites (Joyce and Paykel 1989), several studies have reasonably consistently shown that low urinary MHPG levels predict clinical response to imipramine (Beckman and Goodwin 1975; Fawcett et al. 1972; Garvey et al. 1990; Maas et al. 1984; Mooney et al. 1991). A similar relationship between low urinary MHPG levels and clinical response may also apply to maprotiline (Schatzberg et al. 1981). Results with nortriptyline are mixed, and most studies suggest that urinary MHPG levels do not predict response to amitriptyline (Beckman and Goodwin 1975; Maas et al. 1984; Spiker et al. 1980). Because a substantial portion of urinary MHPG levels may derive from brain metabolites of norepinephrine, these studies suggest that depression marked by relatively low levels of norepinephrine turnover (i.e., low pretreatment urinary MHPG levels) respond well to TCAs, which are somewhat selective for inhibiting norepinephrine uptake at the neuronal synapse (Beckman and Goodwin 1975; Maas et al. 1972; Schildkraut et al. 1986).

Conversely, the measurement of 5-hydroxyindoleacetic acid (5-HIAA) in cerebrospinal fluid may provide an index of cerebral serotonin turnover. There is some evidence that depressed patients with low pretreatment 5-HIAA levels benefit from relatively selective serotonin reuptake blockers such as clomipramine (Van Praag 1977), whereas high 5-HIAA levels may predict better clinical response to amitriptyline (Banki 1977), imipramine (Goodwin and Potter 1978), or nortriptyline (Asberg et al. 1973).

On the basis of studies on psychostimulant response and monoamine metabolites, Maas (1978) suggested that there are two subgroups of depression. The first, which he calls group A, is caused by norepinephrine depletion and is characterized by low urinary MHPG levels, mood-brightening response to psychostimulants, and a clinical response to more noradrenergic TCAs such as imipramine or desipramine. The other subgroup, group B, is a serotonin-deficient depression characterized by normal or high urinary MHPG levels (and presumably low 5-HIAA levels), a dysphoric mood response to amphetamine, and a clinical response to more serotonergic antidepressants such as amitriptyline or clomipramine.

Attractive as the hypothesis of separate norepinephrine and serotonin depressions is, there is little empirical support for it (Joyce and Paykel 1989; Stern et al. 1980). First, there are substantial interactions between the norepinephrine and serotonin receptor symptoms (Potter et al. 1984; Sulser 1987). Second, evidence from plasma level studies suggests that there is considerable overlap among patients who respond to various TCAs as long as adequate doses, as determined by blood levels, are used (Glassman et al. 1977; Kragh-Sorensen et al. 1976).

Enzymes involved in monoamine metabolism. Enzymes have not received much attention as predictors of response to TCAs. One study found that high platelet monoamine oxidase activity predicted response to nortriptyline (Georgotas et al. 1987). Another study found that plasma monoamine oxidase activity was higher in both clomipramine and maprotiline responders than in nonresponders (Fahndrich 1983). Whereas one study suggested that low red blood cell catechol-O-methyltransferase (COMT) levels predicted response to imipramine (Davidson et al. 1976), another found no difference in plasma COMT levels in patients who did or did not respond to clomipramine or maprotiline (Fahndrich 1983).

Precursors of monoamines. The ratio of tyrosine, the amino acid precursor of norepinephrine, to neutral amino acids may predict response to nortriptyline (Moller et al. 1985). Similarly, the ratio of tryptophan—the amino acid precursor of serotonin—to neutral amino acid precursors predicts clinical response to amitriptyline (Moller et al. 1983). Furthermore, tryptophan potentiates TCAs such that depressed mood and anxiety are mollified, but not on the level of psychomotor activity or arousal (Waliner et al. 1976), whereas large doses of L-dopa (a dopamine precursor) lead to improvement in psychomotor retardation, but not in mood (Goodwin et al. 1970). These findings suggest that there might be some relationship between specific amine changes and distinct symptoms or clusters of symptoms (Goodwin et al. 1978), a hypothesis somewhat supported in subsequent studies (Rampello et al. 1991), but not in others (Brotman et al. 1987).

Neuroendocrine challenges. The dexamethasone suppression test (DST) has become the most extensively studied biological test in psychiatry (Ribeiro et al. 1993). One of the earliest questions to emerge in the DST literature concerned its usefulness as a predictor of response to treatment. Reviewing 45 studies that compared treatment response of patients who did and did not suppresss cortisol, Ribeiro and colleagues concluded that pretreatment DST status does not predict short-term response to antidepressant treatment or outcome. On the other hand, patients who do not have suppressed cortisol at baseline do not respond well to placebo, making the TCA-placebo difference larger in this group. Not all of the studies reviewed by Ribeiro's group used TCAs as the only or predominant active treatment; however, TCAs were studied more than any other active treatment or class of antidepressant medication, and the conclusions are the same when considering the 14 studies using only TCAs. Ribeiro and colleagues also reviewed several long-term outcome studies and found that a result of persistent nonsuppression of cortisol on the DST after acute treatment, even if there is clinical improvement, is strongly associated with early relapse or poor outcome. Although there has been some suggestion that cortisol suppression may predict a preferential response to noradrenergic TCAs (Brown and Qualls 1981; Fraser 1983), the majority of studies have not supported this theory (Gitlin and Gerner 1986; Gredan et al. 1981; Joyce and Paykel 1989).

A second neuroendocrine marker that has been used to identify patients with major depression is the thyrotropin-releasing hormone (TRH) stimulation test (Extein et al. 1981), but, as with the DST, questions of specificity and sensitivity have arisen (Loosen and Prange 1982). Although the thyrotropin response to TRH infusion has not yet been found to consistently predict TCA response, a persistently blunted TRH response during antidepressant treatment may be associated with an increased risk of depressive relapse (Kirkegaard 1981; Targum 1984).

Psychophysiologic Measures

Two studies on elderly depressed patients showed that a drop in pretreatment systolic blood pressure of 10 mm Hg or more from supine to standing positions predicted positive response to nortriptyline (Schneider et al. 1986), imipramine, and doxepin (Jarvik et al. 1983), but was not related to any significant orthostatic hypotension during treatment. These observations were replicated and extended by Stack and colleagues (1988) in depressed geriatric inpatients, most of whom also had concurrent medical illness under active treatment. Morning pretreatment systolic blood pressure drop showed a significant inverse correlation with the percent change in Hamilton Depression Rating Scale scores in both nortriptyline, and electroconvulsive therapy–treated patients.

Depressed patients with a shortened REM latency may have a high likelihood of response to TCAs compared with placebo treatment (Coble et al. 1979). Rush and colleagues (1989) found that reduced pretreatment REM latency predicted a positive response in depressed outpatient treatment either with desipramine or with amitriptyline when compared with patients with nonreduced REM latency. REM latency did not differentiate patients who did or did not respond to desipramine or amitriptyline. Kupfer and colleagues (1980) found that during the first few nights of treatment with amitriptyline, patients who eventually had a good therapeutic response to the medication demonstrated greater decreases in the percentage of REM sleep, a greater increase in REM latency, and decreased REM activity compared with nonresponders. Hochli and colleagues (1986) reported similar findings in depressed patients treated with clomipramine. These findings imply a potential clinical role for sleep polysomnography in determining TCA responsiveness. The presence of decreased REM latency would argue for a trial of TCA medication, although choice of a particular TCA may not be assisted by polysomnographic patterns. An early improvement in REM sleep parameters further predicts ultimate response from treatment.

Table 1–2 provides a summary of the probable biological factors that would predict a good response to TCAs.

Conclusion

Fortunately, clinicians now have available to them a number of antidepressant medications besides the tricyclic medications to treat patients with depressive disorders. In many cases, the newer,

Table 1–2. Summary of probable biological predictors of a good response to TCAs

- Mood-brightening response to psychostimulants, especially for imipramine and desipramine
- Low urinary MHPG levels for imipramine (and desipramine) and other purportedly norepinephrine uptake blockers
- Low CSF 5-HIAA levels for amitriptyline (and clomipramine) and other purportedly potent serotonin uptake blockers
- High tyrosine:neutral amino acid ratio for nortriptyline
- High tryptophane:neutral amino acid ratio for amitriptyline
- High platelet or plasma MAO activity
- DST nonsuppression for a robust TCA/placebo difference
- DST suppression after acute treatment for relapse or recurrence
- Normal TRH response after acute treatment for relapse or recurrence
- Pretreatment systolic blood pressure drop ≥10 mm Hg
- Pretreatment shortened REM latency
- Decreased REM sleep after first few days of treatment

Note. MHPG = 3-methoxy-4-hydroxyphenylglycol; CSF 5-HIAA = cerebrospinal fluid level of 5-hydroxyindoleactic acid; DST = dexamethasone suppression test; TRH = thyrotropin-releasing hormone.

nontricyclic agents have more desirable side effect profiles and are less toxic than their forerunners, and increasingly, they are being considered first-line medications by many clinicians. But the TCAs are not dead. They continue to be invaluable agents for the treatment of major depression, dysthymia and other disorders such as subsyndromal depression, anxiety disorders, and pain syndromes.

Since the TCAs are associated with substantial side effects and toxicities, it is important to know which patients are most likely to benefit from them, especially in relation to other possible treatments. The ability to predict optimal response is particularly important in view of the widening spectrums of what are being considered medication response syndromes and the increasing awareness that mood disorders are chronic or recurrent, thus requiring prolonged exposure to potential adverse effects of medication. Unfortunately, there is no consensus regarding predictors of response. The best predictors are probably past response to a particular agent; failing that, the response of a first-degree blood relative might help guide rational decision making. Although severity of depression, melancholic features, or biologic irregularities might not themselves predict response, it is likely that somatic treatment, including TCAs, are particularly indicated in the more severe, melancholic, or biological depressions No single factor absolutely predicts response, but the more indicators for a specific agent that are present, the more likely it is that the patient will respond to that agent.

Although much information is available to clinicians regarding predictors of response to TCAs, more needs to be learned. In particular, it will be important to determine which patients are more likely to respond to TCAs than to the newer agents, to other biological treatment, or to short-term psychotherapies. Under what conditions do TCAs reverse or ameliorate subsyndromal depressions, depressions secondary to adverse life events such as bereavement or divorce, depressions secondary to other medical conditions, or depressions that are comorbid with other psychiatric disorders? We also need better predictors of relapse and recurrence both on and off medications, and more studies of predictors of response at the extremes of age. We now have the available methodology to answer these challenging questions. As the answers emerge, it is likely that TCAs will continue to play a prominent role in the treatment of mood disorders.

References

Abraham HC, Kanter VB, Rosen I, et al: A controlled clinical trial of imipramine (Tofranil) with out-patients. Br J Psychiatry 109:286–293, 1963

Akiskal HS: Factors associated with incomplete recovery in primary depressive illness. J Clin Psychiatry 43:266–271, 1982

Akiskal HS: The bipolar spectrum: new concepts in classification and diagnosis, in Psychiatry Update: The American Psychiatric Association Annual Review, Vol 2. Edited by Grinspoon L. Washington, DC, American Psychiatric Press, 1983, pp 271–292

Akiskal HS: New insights into the nature and heterogeneity of mood disorders. J Clin Psychiatry 50(suppl 5):6–10, 1989

Akiskal HS, Hirschfeld RMA, Yerevanian BI: The relationship of personality to affective disorders: a critical review. Arch Gen Psychiatry 40:801–810, 1983

American Psychiatric Association: Diagnostic and Statistical Manual on Mental Disorders, 3rd Edition. Washington, DC, American Psychiatric Association,1980

American Psychiatric Association: Diagnostic and Statistical Manual on Mental Disorders, 3rd Edition, Revised. Washington, DC, American Psychiatric Association, 1987

American Psychiatric Association: Practice Guideline for Major Depressive Disorder in Adults, 1993

American Psychiatric Association Task Force on the Use of Laboratory Tests in Psychiatry: Tricyclic antidepressants—blood level measurements and clinical outcome: an APA Task Force report. Am J Psychiatry 142:155–162, 1985

Angst J: A clinical analysis of the effects of Tofranil in depression. Psychopharmacologia 2:381–407, 1961

Anton RF, Sexauer JD: Efficacy of amoxapine in psychotic depression. Am J Psychiatry 140:1344–1347, 1983

Asberg M, Bertilsson L, Tuck D, et al: Indoleamine metabolites in cerebrospinal fluid of depressed patients before and during treatment with nortriptyline. Clin Pharmacol Ther 14:277–286, 1973

Banki CM: Correlation of anxiety and related symptoms with cerebrospinal fluid 5-hydroxyindoleacetic acid in depressed women. Journal of Neural Transmission 41:135–143, 1977

Barlow DH, DiNardo PA, Vermilyea DA, et al: Comorbidity and depression among the anxiety disorders. J Nerv Ment Dis 174:63–72, 1986

Beckman H, Goodwin FK: Antidepressant responses to tricyclics and urinary MHPG in unipolar patients. Arch Gen Psychiatry 32:17–21, 1975

Bielski RJ, Friedel RO: Prediction of tricyclic antidepressant response: a critical review. Arch Gen Psychiatry 33:1479–1489, 1976

Black DW, Winokur G, Nasrallah H: Treatment and outcome in secondary depression: a naturalistic study. J Clin Psychiatry 48:438–441, 1987

Black DW, Bell S, Hulbert J, et al: The importance of axis II in patients with major depression. J Affect Disord 14:115–122, 1988

Breier A, Charney DS, Heninger GR: Major depression in panic disorder. Arch Gen Psychiatry 41:1125–1139, 1984

Brockington IF, Helzer JE, Hillier VF, et al: Definition of depression: concordance and prediction of outcome. Am J Psychiatry 139:1022–1027, 1982

Brotman AM, Falk WE, Gelenberg AJ: Pharmacological treatment of acute depressive subtype, in Psychopharmacology: The Third Generation of Progress. Edited by Meltzer HY. New York, Raven Press, 1987, pp 1031–1040

Brown GW, Sklair F, Harris TO, et al: Life events and psychiatric disorders, I: some methodological issues. Psychol Med 3:74–87, 1973

Brown P, Brawley P: Dexamethasone suppression test and mood response to methylphenidate in primary depression. Am J Psychiatry 140:990–993, 1983

Brown WA, Qualls CB: Pituitary-adrenal disinhibition in depression: marker of a subtype with characteristic clinical features and response to treatment? Psychiatry Res 4:115–128, 1981

Bunney WE: The switch process in manic-depressive psychosis. Ann Intern Med 87:319–335, 1977

Caine ED, Lyness JM, King DA, et al: Clinical and etiological heterogeneity of mood disorders in elderly patients, in Diagnosis and Treatment of Depression in Late Life: Results of the NIH Consensus Development Conference. Edited by Schneider LS, Reynolds DF, Lebowitz BD, et al. Washington, DC, American Psychiatric Press, 1994, pp 23–53

Cassano GB, Maggini C, Akiskal HS: Short-term, subchronic, and chronic sequelae of affective disorders. Psychiatr Clin North Am 6:55–67, 1983

Cassem NH: Massachusetts General Hospital Handbook of General Hospital Psychiatry. St Louis, MO, Mosby Year Book, 1991, pp 237–269

Charney DS, Nelson JC: Delusional and nondelusional unipolar depression: further evidence for distinct subtypes. Am J Psychiatry 138:328–333, 1981

Coble PA, Kupfer DJ, Spiker DG, et al: EEG sleep in primary depression: a longitudinal placebo study. J Affect Disord 1:131–138, 1979

Cohen-Cole SA, Stoudemire A: Major depression and physical illness: special considerations in diagnosis and biologic treatment. Psychiatr Clin North Am 10:1–17, 1987

Coryell W, Turner R: Outcome with desipramine therapy in subtypes of nonpsychotic major depression. J Affect Disord 9:149–154, 1985

Coryell W, Coppen A, Zeigler VE, et al: Early improvement as a predictor of response to amitriptyline and nortriptyline: a comparison of 2 patient samples. Psychol Med 12:135–139, 1982

Coryell W, Endicott A, Andreason NC, et al: Depression in panic attacks: the significance of overlap as reflected in follow-up in family study data. Am J Psychiatry 145:293–300, 1988

Davidson JRT, McLeod MN, White HL, et al: Red blood cell catechol o-methyltransferase and response in imipramine in unipolar depressive women. Am J Psychiatry 133:952–955, 1976

Davidson JR, Miller RD, Turnbull CD, et al: Atypical depression. Arch Gen Psychiatry 35:527–534, 1982

Deykin EY, DiMascio A: Relationship of patient background characteristics to efficacy of pharmacotherapy in depression. J Nerv Ment Dis 156:109–129, 1972

Downing RW, Rickels K: Predictors of response to amitriptyline and placebo in three outpatient treatment settings. J Nerv Ment Dis 156:109–120, 1973

Downs NS, Swerdlow NR, Zisook, S: The relationship of affective illness and personality disorders in psychiatric outpatients. Annals of Clinical Psychiatry 4:87–94, 1992

Elkin I, Shea MT, Satkins JT, et al: National Institute of Mental Health Treatment of Depression Collaborative Research Program: general effectiveness of treatments. Arch Gen Psychiatry 46:971–983, 1989

Ettigi PG, Hayes PE, Narasimhacharr N, et al: D-amphetamine response and dexamethasone suppression test as predictors of treatment outcome in unipolar depression. Biol Psychiatry 18:499–504, 1983

Extein I, Pottash A, Gold M: The thyrotropin-releasing hormone test in the diagnosis of unipolar depression. Psychiatry Res 5:311–316, 1981

Faber R, Williams K, Prescott D, et al: Dextroamphetamine and dexamethasone suppression test prediction of desipramine response. Biol Psychiatry 25:654–657, 1989

Fahndrich E: Clinical and biological parameters as predictors for antidepressant drug responses in depressed patients. Pharmacopsychiatry 16:179–185, 1983

Fakhr El-Islam M: Is response to antidepressants an aid to the differentiation of response-specific types of depression? Br J Psychiatry 123:509–511, 1973

Farmer A, McGuffin P: The classification of the depressions: contemporary confusion revisited. Br J Psychiatry 155:437–443, 1989

Fawcett J, Sionopoulos V: Dextroamphetamine response as a possible predictor of improvement with tricyclic therapy in depression. Arch Gen Psychiatry 25:247–255, 1971

Fawcett J, Maas JW, Dekirmenjian H: Depression and MHPG excretion: response to dextroamphetamine and tricyclic antidepressants. Arch Gen Psychiatry 26:246–251, 1972

Feighner JP, Boyer WF: Selective Serotonin Re-uptake Inhibitors: The Clinical Use of Citalopram, Fluoxetine, Fluvoxamine, Paroxetine, and Sertraline. New York, Wiley, 1991

Frank E, Kupfer DJ, Jacob M, et al: Personality features and response to acute treatment in recurrent depression. J Pers Disord 1:14–26, 1987

Frank E, Kupfer DJ, Perel JM, et al: Three-year outcomes for maintenance therapies in recurrent depression. Arch Gen Psychiatry 47:1093–1099, 1990

Frank E, Prien R, Jarrett R, et al: Conceptualization and rationale for consensus definitions of terms in major depressive disorder: response, remission, recovery, relapse and recurrence. Arch Gen Psychiatry 48:851–855, 1991

Fraser AR: Choice of antidepressant based on the dexamethasone suppression test. Am J Psychiatry 140:786–787, 1983

Garvey MJ, Schaffer CB, Tuason VB: Comparison of pharmacological treatment responses between situational and non-situational depressions. Br J Psychiatry 145:353–365, 1984

Garvey M, DeRubeis RJ, Jollon SD, et al: Does 24-hour urinary MHPG predict treatment response to antidepressants? II: association between imipramine response and low MHPG. J Affect Disord 20:181–184, 1990

Georgotas A, McCue RE: The additional benefit of extending an antidepressant trial past 7 weeks in the depressed elderly. International Journal of Geriatric Psychiatry 4:191–195, 1989

Georgotas A, McCue RE, Friedman E, et al: Prediction of response to nortriptyline and phenelzine by platelet MAO activity. Am J Psychiatry 144:338–340, 1987

Georgotas A, McCue RE, Cooper TB, et al: Factors affecting the delay of antidepressant effect in responders to nortriptyline and phenelzine. Psychiatry Res 28:1–9, 1989

Gerson SC, Plotkin DA, Jarvik LF: Antidepressant drug studies, 1964–1986: empirical evidence for aging patients. J Clin Psychopharmacol 8:311–322, 1988

Gitlin MJ, Gerner RH: The dexamethasone suppression test and response to somatic treatment: a review. J Clin Psychiatry 47:16–21, 1986

Glassman AH, Roose SP: Delusional depression: a distinct clinical entity? Arch Gen Psychiatry 38:424–427, 1981

Glassman AH, Perel JM, Shostak M, et al: Clinical implications of imipramine plasma levels for depressive illness. Arch Gen Psychiatry 34:197–204, 1977

Goodwin FK, Potter WZ: The biology of affective illness: amine neurotransmitters and drug response, in Depression: Biology, Psychodynamics, and Treatment. Edited by Cole JO, Schatzberg AF, Frazier SH. New York, Plenum, 1978

Goodwin FK, Brodie HKH, Murphy DL, et al: L-Dopa, catecholamines and behavior: a clinical and biochemical study in depressed patients. Biol Psychiatry 2:341–366, 1970

Goodwin FK, Cowdry RW, Webster MH: Predictors of drug response in the affective disorders: toward an integrated approach, in Psychopharmacology: A Generation of Progress. Edited by Lipton MA, DiMascio A, Killam KF. New York, Raven, 1978, pp 1278–1288

Gredan J, Kronfol Z, Gardner R, et al: Dexamethasone suppression test and selection of antidepressant medications. J Affect Disord 3:389–396, 1981

Grunhaus L, Rabin D, Gredan JF: Simultaneous panic and depressive disorder: response to antidepressant treatment. J Clin Psychiatry 47:4–7, 1986

Grunhaus L, Harel Y, Krugler T, et al: Major depressive disorder and panic disorder: effects of comorbidity on treatment outcome with antidepressant medications. Clin Neuropharmacol 5:454–461, 1988

Hirschfeld RMA, Klerman GL, Andreasen NC, et al: Psychosocial predictors of chronicity in depressed patients. Br J Psychiatry 148:648–654, 1986

Hochli D, Riemann D, Zuley J, et al: Initial REM sleep suppression by clomipramine: a prognostic tool for treatment response in patients with a major depressive disorder. Biol Psychiatry 21:1217–1220, 1986

Hodern A, Holt NF, Burt CG, et al: Amitriptyline in depressive states, phenomenology and prognostic considerations. Br J Psychiatry 109:815–825, 1963

Himmelhoch JM, Thase ME, Mallinger AG, et al: Tranylcypromine versus imipramine in anergic bipolar depression. Am J Psychiatry 148:910–916, 1991.

Jarvik LF, Mintz J, Steuer J, et al: Treating geriatric depression: a 26-week interim analysis. J Am Geriatr Soc 30:713–717, 1982

Jarvik LF, Read SL, Mintz J, et al: Pretreatment orthostatic hypotension in geriatric depression: predictor of response to imipramine and doxepin. J Clin Psychopharmacol 3:368–372, 1983.

Jenike MA: Treatment of affective illness in the elderly with drugs and electroconvulsive therapy. J Geriatr Psychiatry 22:77–112, 1989

Joffe RT, Regan JJ: Personality and response to tricyclic antidepressants in depressed patients. J Nerv Ment Dis 177:745–749, 1989

Joyce PR, Paykel ES: Predictors of drug response in depression. Arch Gen Psychiat 46:89–99, 1989

Kantor SJ, Glassman AH: Delusional depressions: natural history and response to treatment. Br J Psychiatry 131:351–360, 1977

Katon W, Sullivan MD: Depression and chronic medical illness. J Clin Psychiatry 51(suppl):3–11, 1991

Katz IR, Simpson GM, Curlik SM, et al: Pharmacologic treatment of major depression for elderly patients in residential care settings. J Clin Psychiatry 51(suppl):41–47, 1990

Katz MM, Koslow SH, Maas JW, et al: The timing, specificity and clinical prediction of tricyclic drug effects in depression. Psychol Med 17:297–309, 1987

Keller MB, Klerman GL, Lavori PW, et al: Treatment received by depressed patients. JAMA 248:1848–1855, 1982

Keller MB, Lavori PW, Coryell W, et al: Differential outcome of pure manic, mixed/cycling and pure depressive episodes in patients with bipolar illness. JAMA 255:3138–3142, 1986a

Keller MB, Lavori PW, Rice J, et al: The persistent risk of chronicity in recurrent episodes of nonbipolar major depressive disorder: a prospective follow-up. Am J Psychiatry 143:24–28, 1986b

Keller MB, Lavori PW, Mueller TI, et al: Time to recovery, chronicity, and levels of psychopathology in major depression. Arch Gen Psychiatry 49:809–816, 1992

Kendall RE: The classification of depressions: a review of contemporary confusion. Br J Psychiatry 129:15–28, 1976

Kiloh LG, Ball JRB, Garside RF: Prognostic factors in treatment of depressive states with imipramine. BMJ 1:1225–1227, 1962

Kirkegaard C: The thyrotropin response to thyrotropin-releasing hormone in endogenous depression. Psychoneuroendocrinology 6:189–212, 1981

Klein DF: Endogenomorphic depression. Arch Gen Psychiatry 31:447–454, 1974

Klein DF, Davis JM: Diagnosis and drug treatment of psychiatric disorders. Baltimore, MD, Williams and Wilkins, 1980, pp 379–390

Kocis JH, Croughan JL, Katz MM, et al: Response to treatment with antidepressants of patients with severe or moderate nonpsychotic depression and of patients with psychotic depression. Am J Psychiatry 147:621–624, 1990

Kragh-Sorensen P, Hansen CE, Baastrup PC: Relationship between antidepressant effect and plasma level of nortriptyline: clinical studies. Pharmakopsychiatr Neuropsychopharmakol 9:27–32, 1976

Kupfer DJ, Spiker DG. Refractory depression: prediction of nonresponse by clinical indicators. J Clin Psychiatry 42:307–312, 1981

Kupfer DJ, Spiker DG, Coble PA, et al: Depression, EEG sleep, and clinical response. Compr Psychiatry 21:212–220, 1980

Kupfer DJ, Frank E, Perel JM, et al: Five-year outcome for maintenance therapies in recurrent depression. Arch Gen Psychiatry 49:769–773, 1992

Leibowitz HR, Quitkin FM, Stewart JW, et al: Antidepressant specificity in atypical depression. Arch Gen Psychiatry 45:129–137, 1988

Lloyd C, Zisook S, Click M, et al: Life events and response to antidepressants. Journal of Human Stress 7:2–16, 1981

Loyd DW, Tsuang MT: Duration criteria and long-term outcome in affective disorder and schizophrenia. J Affect Disord 9:35–39, 1985

Loosen PT, Prange AJ: Serum thyrotropin response to thyroid-releasing hormone in psychiatric patients: a review. Am J Psychiatry 139:405–416, 1982

Lydiard RB: Tricyclic-resistant depression: treatment resistance or inadequate treatment? J Clin Psychiatry 46:412–417, 1985

Lydiard RB: Coexisting depression and anxiety: special diagnostic and treatment issues. J Clin Psychiatry 52(suppl 6):48–54, 1991

Maas JW: Clinical and biochemical heterogeneity of depressive disorders. Ann Intern Med 88:556–563, 1978

Maas JW, Fawcett JA, Dekirmenjian H: Catecholamine metabolism, depressive illness, and drug response. Arch Gen Psychiatry 26:252–262, 1972

Maas JW, Koslow SH, Katz MM, et al: Pretreatment neurotransmitter metabolite levels and response to tricyclic antidepressant drugs. Am J Psychiatry 141:1159–1171, 1984

McGrath PJ, Stewart JW, Harrison WM, et al: Predictive value of symptoms of atypical depression for differential drug treatment outcome. J Clin Psychopharmacol 12:197–202, 1992

Moller SE, Honore P, Larsen OB: Tryptophan and tyrosine ratios to neutral amino acids in endogenous depression: relation to antidepressant response to amitriptyline and lithium/L-tryptophan. J Affect Disord 5:67–79, 1983

Moller SE, Odum K, Kirk L, et al: Plasma tyrosine/neutral amino acid ration correlated with clinical response to nortriptyline in endogenously depressed patients. J Affect Disord 9:223–229, 1985

Mooney JJ, Schatzberg AF, Cole JO, et al: Urinary 3-methoxy-4-hydroxyphenylglycol and the depression-type score as predictors of differential responses to antidepressants. J Clin Psychopharmacol 11:339–343, 1991

Nagayama H, Nagano K, Ikezaki A, et al: Prediction of efficacy of antidepressant by 1-week test therapy in depression. J Affect Disord 23:213–216, 1991

Nelson JC, Mazure CM, Jatlow PI: Does melancholia predict response in major depression? J Affect Disord 18:157–165, 1990

Nelson JC, Mazure CM, Jatlow PI: Characteristics of desipramine-refractory depression. J Clin Psychiatry 55:12–19, 1994

Pare CMB, Mack JW: Differentiation of two genetically specific types of depression by the response to antidepressant drugs. J Med Genet 8:306–309, 1971

Paykel ES: Depressive typologies and response to amitriptyline. Br J Psychiatry 120:147–156, 1972

Paykel ES, Myers JK, Dienelt MN, et al: Life events and depression: a controlled study. Arch Gen Psychiatry 21:753–760, 1969

Paykel ES, Prusoff BA, Klerman GL, et al: Clinical response to amitriptyline among depressed women. J Nerv Ment Dis 156:149–165, 1973

Paykel ES, Rowan PR, Parker RR, et al: Response to phenelzine and amitriptyline in subtypes of outpatient depressives. Arch Gen Psychiatry 39:1041–1049, 1982

Peselow ED, Sanfilipo MP, Difiglia C, et al: Melancholic/endogenous depression and response to somatic treatment and placebo. Am J Psychiatry 149:1324–1334, 1992

Pfohl B, Stangl D, Zimmerman M: The implications of DSM-III personality disorders for patients with major depression. J Affect Disord 7:309–318, 1984

Pilkonis PA, Frank EL: Personality pathology in recurrent depression: nature, prevalence, and relationship to treatment response. Am J Psychiatry 145:435–441, 1988

Popkin MK, Callies AL, Mackenzie TB: The outcome of antidepressant use in the medically ill. Arch Gen Psychiatry 42:1160–1163, 1985

Potter WZ, Karoum F, Linnoila M: Common mechanism of action of biochemically "specific" antidepressants. Prog Neuropsychopharmacol Biol Psychiatry 8:152–161, 1984

Prusoff BA, Weissman MM, Klerman GL, et al: Research diagnostic criteria subtypes of depression. Arch Gen Psychiatry 37:796–801, 1980

Quadri AA, Shalini K, Channabasavanna SM: Amphetamine as a predictor for response to imipramine and amitriptyline. Indian J Psychiatry 22:182–194, 1980

Quitkin FM, Rabkin J, Ross D, et al: Identification of response to antidepressants. Arch Gen Psychiatry 41:782–786, 1984

Quitkin FM, Rabkin JD, Markowitz JM, et al: Use of pattern analysis to identify true drug response. Arch Gen Psychiatry 44:259–264, 1987

Quitkin FM, Stewart JW, McGrath P, et al: Phenelzine versus imipramine in the treatment of probable atypical depression: defining syndrome boundaries of selective MAOI responders. Am J Psychiatry 145:306–312, 1988

Quitkin FM, Harrison W, Stewart JW, et al: Response to phenelzine and imipramine in placebo nonresponders with atypical depression: a new application of the crossover design. Arch Gen Psychiatry 48:319–323, 1991

Rampello L, Nicoletti G, Raffaele R: Dopaminergic hypothesis for retarded depression: a symptom profile for predicting therapeutical responses. Acta Psychiatr Scand 84:552–554, 1991

Raskin A: Age-sex differences in response to antidepressant drugs. J Nerv Ment Dis 159:120–130, 1974

Raskin A, Crook TH: The endogenous-neurotic distinction as a predictor of response to antidepressant drugs. Psychol Med 6:59–70, 1976

Raskin A, Schulterbrandt JG, Boothe H: Treatment, social and psychiatric history variables related to symptom reduction in hospitalized depression, in Psychopharmacology and the Individual Patient. Edited by Wittenborn JR, Goldberg SC, May PRA. New York, Raven Press, 1970, pp 135–159

Reich JH, Vasile RG: Effect of personality disorders on the treatment outcome of Axis I conditions: an update. J Nerv Ment Dis 181:475–484, 1993

Reynolds CF, Frank E, Perel JM, et al: Treatment of consecutive episodes of major depression in the elderly. Am J Psychiatry 151:1740–1743, 1994

Ribeiro SCM, Tandon R, Grunhaus L, et al: The DST as a predictor of outcome in depression: a meta-analysis. Am J Psychiatry 150:1618–1629, 1993

Richelson E: Biological basis of depression and therapeutic relevance. J Clin Psychiatry 52(suppl 6):4–10, 1991

Rickels K, Ward CH, Schut L: Different populations, different drug responses. Am J Med Sci 247:328–335, 1964

Robinson DS, Kayser A, Corcella J, et al: Panic attacks in outpatients with depression: response to treatment. Psychopharmacol Bull 21:562–567, 1985

Roose SP, Glassman AH, Walsh BT, et al: Tricyclic nonresponders, phenomenology and treatment. Am J Psychiatry 143:345–348, 1986

Rush AJ, Roffwarg HP, Giles DE, et al: Psychobiological predictors of antidepressant drug response. Pharmacopsychiatrica 16:192–194, 1983

Rush JA, Giles DE, Jarrett RB, et al: Reduced REM latency predicts response to tricyclic medication in depressed outpatients. Biol Psychiatry 26:61–72, 1989

Sabelli HC, Fawcett J, Javid JJ, et al: The methylphenidate test for differentiating desipramine responsive from nortriptyline responsive depression. Am J Psychiatry 140:212–214, 1983

Salzman C: Pharmacological treatment of depression in elderly patients, in Diagnosis and Treatment of Depression in Late Life: Results of the NIH Consensus Development Conference. Edited by Schneider LS, Reynolds CF, Lebowitz BD, et al. Washington, DC, American Psychiatric Press, 1994, pp 181–244

Schatzberg AF: Dosing strategies for antidepressant agents. J Clin Psychiatry 52(suppl):14–20, 1991

Schatzberg AF, Rosenbaum AH, Orsulak PJ, et al: Toward a biochemical classification of depressive disorders, III: pretreatment urinary MHPG levels as predictors of response to treatment with maprotiline. Psychopharmacology 75:34–38, 1981

Schatzberg AF, Cole JO, Cohen BM, et al: Survey of depressed patients who have failed to respond to treatment, in The Affective Disorders. Edited by Davis JM, Maas JW. Washington, DC, American Psychiatric Press, 1983

Schildkraut JJ, Schatzberg AF, Mooney JJ, et al: Toward a biochemical classification of depressive disorders: differential responses to treatment, in Proceedings of the IVth World Congress of Biological Psychiatry. Edited by Shagrass C, et al. New York, Elsevier, 1986, pp 16–18

Schneider LS, Sloane RB, Staples FR, et al: Pretreatment orthostatic hypotension as a predictor of response to nortriptyline in geriatric depression. J Clin Psychopharmacol 6:172–176, 1986

Shawcross CR, Tyrer P: Influence of personality on response to monoamine oxidase inhibitors and tricyclic antidepressants. J Psychiatr Res 19:557–562, 1985

Shea MT, Pilkonis PA, Beckham E, et al: Personality disorders and treatment outcome in the NIMH treatment of depression collaborative research program. Am J Psychiatry 147:711–718, 1990

Simpson GM, Lee JH, Cuculic A, et al: Two dosages of imipramine in hospitalized endogenous and neurotic depressives. Arch Gen Psychiatry 33:1093–1102, 1976

Sorensen B, Kragh-Sorensen P, Larsen NE, et al: The practical significance of nortriptyline plasma control: a prospective evaluation under routine conditions in endogenous depression. Psychopharmacology 59:35–39, 1978

Sotsky SM, Glass DR, Shea MT, et al: Patient predictors of response to psychotherapy and pharmacology: findings in the NIMH treatment of depression collaborative research program. Am J Psychiatry 148:997–1008, 1991

Spar JA, La Rue A: Acute response to methylphenidate as a predictor of outcome of treatment with TCAs in the elderly. J Clin Psychiatry 46:466–469, 1985

Spiker PG, Edwards D, Hanin I, et al: Urinary MHPG and clinical response to amiptriptyline in depressed patients. Am J Psychiatry 137:1183–1187, 1980

Spiker DS, Weiss JC, Dealy RS, et al: The pharmacological treatment of delusional depression. Am J Psychiatry 142:430–436, 1985

Stack JA, Reynolds CF, Perel JM, et al: Pretreatment systolic orthostatic blood pressure and treatment response in elderly depressed inpatients. J Clin Psychopharmacol 8:116–120, 1988

Stern SL, Rush AJ, Mendels J: Toward a rational pharmacology of depression. Am J Psychiatry 137:545–552, 1980

Stewart JW, Quitkin F, Liebowitz MR, et al: Efficacy of desipramine in depressed outpatients. Arch Gen Psychiatry 40:202–207, 1983

Sulser F: Serotonin-norepinephrine receptor interactions in the brain: implications for the pharmacology and pathophysiology of affective disorders. J Clin Psychiatry 48(suppl):12–18, 1987

Targum SD: Persistent neuroendocrine dysregulation in major depressive disorder: a marker for early relapse. Biol Psychiatry 19:305–318, 1984

Thase ME, Carpenter L, Kupfer DJ, et al: Atypical depression: diagnostic and pharmacologic controversies. Psychopharmacol Bull 27:17–22, 1991

Thase ME, Frank E, Mallinger AG, et al: Treatment of imipramine-resistant recurrent depression. III: Efficacy of monoamine oxidase inhibitors. J Clin Psychiatry 53:5–11, 1992.

Thompson LW, Gallagher D, Czirr R: Personality disorder and outcome in the treatment of late-life depression. J Geriatr Psychiatry 21:133–153, 1988

van Kammen DP, Murphy DL: Prediction of imipramine antidepressant response by a 1-day *d*-amphetamine trial. Am J Psychiatry 135:1179–1184, 1978

Van Praag HM: New evidence of serotonin deficient depressions. Neuropsychobiology 3:56–63, 1977

Vollrath M, Angst A: Outcome of panic and depression in a 7-year follow-up: results of the Zurich Study. Acta Psychiatr Scand 80:591–599, 1989

Waliner J, Skott A, Carlsson A, et al: Potentiation of the antidepressant action of clomipramine by tryptophan. Arch Gen Psychiatry 33:1384–1389, 1976

Wehr TA, Goodwin FK: Can antidepressants cause mania and worsen course of affective illness? Am J Psychiatry 144:1403–1411, 1987

Weissman MM, Prusoff BA, Klerman GL, et al: Personality and the prediction of long-term outcome of depression. Am J Psychiatry 135:797–800, 1978

Wells KB, Golding JM, Burnam MA. Psychiatric disorder in a sample of the general population with and without chronic medical conditions. Am J Psychiatry 145:976–981, 1988

Wells KB, Burnam MA, Rogers W, et al: The course of depression in adult outpatients. Arch Gen Psychiatry 49:788–794, 1992

Wittenborn JR, Kiremitei N, Weber E: The choice of alternative antidepressants. J Nerv Ment Dis 156:97–108, 1973

Zimmerman M, Spitzer RL: Melancholia: from DSM-III to DSM-III-R. Am J Psychiatry 146:20–28, 1989

Zimmerman M, Coryell W, Pfohl BM: The treatment validity of DSM-III melancholic subtyping. Psychiatry Res 16:37–43, 1985

Zimmerman M, Coryell W, Pfohl B: The validity of four definitions of endogenous depression, II: clinical, demographic, familial and psychosocial correlates. Arch Gen Psychiatry 43:1090–1096, 1986

Zisook S: A clinical overview of monoamine oxidase inhibitors. Psychosomatics 26:240–251, 1985

Zisook S, Andia AM: Pharmacotherapy of major depression in the 1990s. Hospital Formulary 27:332–353, 1992

Zisook S, Jaffe K, Click M, et al: Rapid responders to tricyclic antidepressants. Journal of Psychiatric Treatment and Evaluation 4:73–80, 1982

Zisook S, Shuchter SR, Gallagher T, et al: Atypical depression in an outpatient psychiatric population. Depression 1:268–274, 1993

CHAPTER 2

Monoamine Oxidase Inhibitors

Raymond Ownby, M.D.,
and Paul J. Goodnick, M.D.

*M*onoamine oxidase inhibitors (MAOIs) were introduced in the 1950s for the treatment of depression. Although they were found to be clearly effective in the treatment of various types of depression, concerns about the possibility of important unwanted effects have limited their use. The most serious of these effects is the development of hypertensive crisis. Because all of the originally introduced MAOIs are irreversible inhibitors of monoamine oxidase—in contrast to the newer reversible MAOIs—the possibility exists that if a patient eats foods containing tyramine, an excess of noradrenergic transmitters can lead to dangerous elevations of blood pressure. This may be a manageable risk in patients who conscientiously eliminate tyramine-containing foods from their diet. When MAOIs are indicated, many clinicians prescribe them for patients who are likely to comply with these dietary restrictions.

More recently, there has been renewed interest in MAOIs because of suggestions that they may be particularly effective for some subtypes of depression as well as other diagnoses, such as panic disorder or borderline personality disorder. An even newer development is the reversible inhibitor of monoamines (RIMA). These medications do not cause long-term inhibition of monoamine oxidase and are unlikely to cause tyramine-related hypertensive crises. In this chapter we review the status of knowledge on the prediction of response to MAOIs in major depression.

Clinical and behavioral predictors are discussed first, followed by biological and pharmacological predictors.

Clinical and Behavioral Predictors

Various clinical features predict a positive response to MAOIs prescribed for depression. Among them are *atypical depression* with reversed vegetative signs (hyperphagia, hypersomnia) and *anergic bipolar* depression. Failure to respond to tricyclic antidepressants (TCAs) may be regarded as a relative predictor of a positive response to MAOIs, according to data that show that in a number of cases in which TCAs failed to bring about a response, patients subsequently responded to MAOIs (Thase et al. 1992b).

Bipolar Depression

There have been a number of reports on the use of MAOIs in bipolar depression. In the earliest study, Himmelhoch and colleagues (1972) reported results of an open trial of tranylcypromine with 21 "depressed patients with bipolar characteristics," including anergia, hypersomnia, and retardation. Despite the overall bipolar description, only 13 patients were found to be bipolar; the other 8 were unipolar. Patients received a mean dose of 30 mg/day of tranylcypromine, and 16 of the 21 (76%) had a "good to excellent" response. Unfortunately, no data in the form of Hamilton Depression Rating Scale (HDRS) or Beck Depression Inventory (BDI) scores were provided. Four of the five patients with an inadequate response had been diagnosed as "schizoaffective" in the past. The follow-up to this study (Himmelhoch et al. 1982) included a sample of 59 depressed patients, 40 of whom were bipolar and showed a 71% response to tranylcypromine.

The most recent report by Himmelhoch and colleagues (1991) concerned the response of 56 patients who met the criteria for major depression associated with a history of bipolar disorder as defined in DSM-III and Research Diagnostic Criteria (RDC). According to the RDC, 43% were bipolar I (associated with history of mania), and 57% were bipolar II (associated with hypomania). All patients were also experiencing hypersomnia or had experienced weight gain.

In this double-blind study, patients were randomly assigned

dosages of a mean of either 36.8 mg of tranylcypromine or 245.5 mg of imipramine per day for an initial period of 6 weeks, followed by a continuation phase of 10 weeks. Among the patients who completed 4 weeks of active treatment, significant response was evaluated by a moderate or marked improvement on the Clinical Global Inventory (CGI), sustained for at least 2 weeks by week 6 or the endpoint. The result was significantly better for tranylcypromine (21/26, 81%) than for imipramine (10/21, 48%) ($P = .02$). Furthermore, of 12 patients who did not respond to imipramine, 9 (75%) then showed significant improvement when given tranylcypromine. In the reverse scenario, only one of four patients who did not respond to tranylcypromine (25%) responded to imipramine (Thase et al. 1992b).

Atypical Depression

In an article often credited as the first to define *atypical depression*, Davidson and colleagues (1982) reviewed how the concept was developed as well as the studies relating to its treatment. The article stated that the London group (St. Thomas Hospital and other centers) reported that MAOIs were the preferred therapy in patients with "anxiety, tension, phobias, panic, hysterical features, irritability, mood reactivity, overeating, oversleeping, and increased libido." It was later reported that such patients should be divided into groups with rejection-sensitive hysteroid dysphoria and those with panic-phobic disorder (Quitkin et al. 1979). Davidson's group then suggested that MAOI-responsive patients be classified as "A" for anxious and "V" for vegetative subtypes. After reviewing the available minimal evidence of differential responsiveness to MAOIs in these disorders, they tentatively concluded that there was modest evidence to support the use of MAOIs in patients with the better-defined entity of "atypical depression."

McGrath and colleagues (1987) studied the outpatient treatment of depressed patients who did not respond to initial phase I interventions with imipramine, phenelzine, or placebo. All patients met RDC criteria for major, minor, or intermittent depression. The patients, however, were required to be "mood reactive" (i.e., able to experience a mood lift from favorable stimuli, a core feature of atypical depression). In a double-blind study, the patients were crossed over to further treatment in phases II and III, each 6 weeks in length. They were treated with a maximum of either 90 mg/day of phenelzine or 300 mg/day of imipramine in each 6-week phase. It was found that of the phase I placebo non-responders, 56% responded to phenelzine and 44% to imipramine in phase II, whereas 88% responded to phenelzine and 20% to imipramine in phase III. Fifty-nine percent of phase I patients who did not respond to imipramine responded to phenelzine in phase II, whereas only 33% of phase I patients who did not respond to phenelzine responded to imipramine in phase II. Thus, the trait of mood reactivity distinguished patients who responded to phenelzine from those who responded to imipramine. McGrath's group concluded that "nonendogenously depressed outpatients who do not respond to vigorous outpatient tricyclic treatment should receive a trial of phenelzine and have a very good chance of responding to it" (p. 171).

In 1989, Quitkin et al. presented results of a study with 60 patients with RDC for major, intermittent, or minor depressive disorder. They studied only those patients diagnosed with simple mood-reactive depression because the phenelzine and imipramine responses had already been shown in both definite atypical depression with at least two associated symptoms of hyperphagia, hypersomnia, leaden feeling, and rejection sensitivity (Liebowitz et al. 1988), and in probable atypical depression (PAD) with one associated symptom (Quitkin et al. 1988). Patients were treated with a maximum of 90 mg/day of phenelzine or 300 mg/day of imipramine for 6 weeks. Response was defined as a rating of 1 (very much improved) or 2 (much improved) on the 7-point CGI. In contrast to the results of the definite atypical depression group and probable atypical depression group, in which the response to phenelzine (71%) was greater than that of imipramine (49%), patients with simple mood-reactive depression in both groups showed a significant response: 75% for phenelzine and 74% for imipramine. A subsequent study from the same group (Stewart et al. 1989) contrasted the responses to phenelzine, imipramine, and placebo among 194 patients who met the criteria for DSM-III major depression or dysthymic disorder with symptoms of probable atypical depression. Maximum dosages and periods of treatment were the same as in the group's previous study. This study yielded similar results to the previous one. There were many more responders among phenelzine patients

(71%) than either imipramine (48%) or placebo patients (26%); however, the difference between phenelzine and imipramine was more pronounced in major depression (75% versus 37%). In dysthymic disorder, imipramine patients (78%) fared somewhat better than phenelzine patients (58%).

Because a reexamination of the data obtained by Liebowitz and colleagues (1988) indicated that the superiority of imipramine and phenelzine to placebo had appeared to be "limited" to those patients with "spontaneous panic attacks and/or hysteroid dysphoria (i.e., rejection hypersensitivity)," a second trial was conducted in an attempt to determine if panic attacks were a contributing predictor to response to medication. Quitkin and colleagues (1990) assembled another sample of 90 patients with atypical depression and contrasted the outcome with the original 120 patients in the Liebowitz study. The replication group with definite atypical depression again showed phenelzine and imipramine responses of 83% and 50%, respectively. This replication attempt indicated that a past history of panic attack was not related to outcome.

Thase and colleagues (1991) completed a study of 211 outpatients with major depression according to DSM-III and RDC. Patients who did not respond to either imipramine or interpersonal psychotherapy received a 6-week open trial with an MAOI (phenelzine $n = 4$, tranylcypromine $n = 36$). Response was defined as a reduction of 50% on the HDRS score. Patients with reversed vegetative signs responded particularly well to MAOIs, whether mood reactive (6/6, 100%) or mood nonreactive (15/21, 71%), as opposed to patients with "typical depression" (5/13, 38%). In a further elaboration of this study, five variables thought to relate to a more favorable response to MAOIs were tested: female sex, younger age, higher pre-MAOI depression scores, poorer prior response to imipramine and interpersonal psychotherapy, and higher pre-MAOI Reverse Vegetative Symptom Scale (RVSS) score (Thase et al. 1992a). With a final mean dose of 60 mg/day for phenelzine and 38.5 mg/day for tranylcypromine, there was a mean overall reduction of 52% on the HDRS score. Treatment response was positive in previous nonresponders to either lithium or thyroid adjunctive trials. As predicted, there were significant positive correlations between percent change on HDRS score and pre-MAOI HDRS score ($r = .36$, $P < .05$), and between post-

and pre-MAOI RVSS scores ($r = .38$, $P < .02$). As anticipated, improvement during treatment with imipramine and interpersonal psychotherapy was inversely related to change during MAOI therapy ($r = -.35$, $P < .05$). Neither sex nor age was associated with MAOI response. In terms of practical application, 87% of responders had two of three subtype diagnoses of atypical or anergic depression (RVSS ≥ 5) and a response to treatment with imipramine and interpersonal psychotherapy of less than 25%. These same results were found in only 47% of nonresponders ($P < .02$).

A summary review of the clinical results of participants in the earlier studies was presented by McGrath and colleagues (1992). This analysis of 401 patients was aimed at determining 1) which features of atypical depression were particularly predictive of outcome, 2) if greater numbers of atypical depression symptoms were more strongly predictive, and 3) in terms of outcome relevance, if "atypical" depression was due primarily to the absence of "typical" symptoms. Results indicated only that oversleeping and leaden paralysis were less predictive of response to imipramine; however, no particular symptom was more predictive of response to phenelzine. The researchers also found that two symptoms of atypical depression more accurately predicted a positive response to phenelzine than did one symptom. In terms of endogenicity being a negative predictor or response to phenelzine, no such symptoms were specifically associated with a better response to imipramine than to phenelzine.

Nolen and colleagues (1988) reported on the effectiveness of tranylcypromine in depressed patients who had previously been unresponsive to at least two other treatments. Eighty-nine patients were enrolled in the first phase of the study; all of these patients had been unsuccessfully treated with adequate tricyclic antidepressant therapy, met DSM-III criteria for major depression, and had a minimum 17-item HDRS score of 18. Of the 89 patients, only those who were subsequently nonresponsive to either oxaprotiline or fluvoxamine and to subsequent sleep deprivation were placed in a randomized open treatment design with either L-5-hydroxytryptophan (L-5-HTP) or tranylcypromine. Overall, 25 of 50 tranylcypromine patients (50%) showed response as defined by a reduction in HDRS score of 50% or more. This response lasted a minimum of 6 months. Sixteen patients (32%) showed an initial response to phenelzine followed by relapse, and nine (18%) showed absolutely no response to phenelzine. Major differences in the characteristics of patients who responded to treatment and patients who did not respond to treatment at all related to the higher endogenous attributes and to a reduced duration of illness in the patients who responded.

The Columbia group presented data of a similar style based on previous groups of patients showing no response to alternate treatments: patients who did not respond to imipramine were switched to phenelzine, and patients who did not respond to phenelzine were switched to imipramine (McGrath et al. 1993). All patients were mood reactive (part of atypical depression) and met the criteria for RDC major, intermittent, or minor depression. Of 89 patients that were crossed over, 72% had major depression, 46% had intermittent depression, 13% had bipolar II disorder, 51% had definite atypical depression, and 26% had probable atypical depression. Results showed that 21 of the 41 patients (51%) who switched from imipramine to phenelzine responded, and eight of the 25 patients (32%) who switched from phenelzine to imipramine responded. Of the patients who did not respond to placebo, those subsequently switched to phenelzine responded better than patients who were subsequently switched to imipramine (55% versus 27%, respectively; $P = .01$). McGrath's group concluded that "under controlled double-blind conditions, relatively chronically depressed, mood-reactive outpatients with atypical symptoms who are unresponsive to treatment with tricyclic antidepressants, show a clinically significant rate of response to MAOIs" (p. 122).

Case 1: Atypical depression. A 58-year old man presented with a chief complaint of depression and lack of interest. His significant symptoms of major depression were hypersomnia, fatigue (leaden paralysis), loss of social interest, lack of motivation, loss of concentration, and loss of libido. He had previously been seen at a major medical clinic and given treatment for back pain. His thyroid tests were within normal limits. He had been an engineer but had to stop working because of increased fatigue.

He had undergone treatment with amoxapine, imipramine, desipramine, and trazodone. All of these treatments lasted several weeks, were of little antidepressive benefit to the patient, and caused various disabling side effects; for example, trazodone caused him to fall asleep while driving, and desipramine caused dry mouth, constipation, jitters, and problems with urination.

He was administered up to 80 mg/day of fluoxetine, which led to increased agitation but had no antidepressive benefit. Due to his lack of response to or tolerance of other standard antidepressants, the patient was given 15 mg of phenelzine twice a day. Before treatment, his BDI score was 39, indicating significant depression. After 8 days, the dose was doubled to 60 mg/day. After 22 days, his BDI score had dropped by over 50%–18. During therapy the BDI score improved gradually to 13, and he became more productive and required less sleep. Unfortunately, the phenelzine later had to be discontinued because, at antidepressant-effective doses, the patient experienced excessive daytime drowsiness, particularly while driving.

Moclobemide

Moclobemide is representative of RIMAs as a drug class. This medication is available in Canada and may soon be approved for distribution in the United States. RIMAs seem to lack three of the most serious complications of standard MAOI use: hepatoxicity, tyramine-induced hypertensive reaction, and orthostatic hypotension (Da Prada et al. 1990). One study in which 2,300 patients were given doses of moclobemide of up to 600 mg/day with no dietary restrictions reported few side effects and no tyramine hypertensive reactions (Versiani et al. 1990). In terms of efficacy in major depression, Versiani and colleagues (1989) contrasted response in a 6-week trial of 300–600 mg/day of moclobemide, 100–200 mg/day of imipramine, or placebo. Moclobemide was equally as effective as imipramine in endogenous depression (51% versus 52% reduction in HDRS score) but slightly less effective in reactive/neurotic depression (45% versus 53% reduction in HDRS score). Biziere and Berger (1990) contrasted response in two studies of 353 patients receiving 300–600 mg/day of moclobemide and 356 patients receiving 100–200 mg/day of imipramine. Patients met DSM-III criteria for major depression and were further classified by ICD-9 into endogenous or reactive subtypes. Response was determined by a reduction of at least 50% on the HDRS score. Results were similar for endogenous depression for moclobemide and imipramine (65% and 67% response, respectively). In reactive depression, however, the rate of response to moclobemide was lower than that to imipramine (58% versus 66%). For both moclobemide and imipramine, response rates were greater in patients age 60 years or younger (both 62%) than for patients age 60 years (51% and 48%, respectively).

Lecrubier and Guelfi (1990) presented a summary of three studies of moclobemide versus imipramine and placebo. A total of 763 patients with DSM-III major depression were in multicenter, double-blind, randomized trials. In the first study, mean dosing after 3 weeks was 510 mg/day of moclobemide and 160 mg/day of imipramine. Over 6 weeks of treatment, the reduction in HDRS score was 52% for moclobemide and 56% for imipramine, both significantly better than the 29% for placebo. Response in endogenous depression was also similar: 50.9% for moclobemide, 51.7% for imipramine. The second trial compared a mean of 476 mg/day of moclobemide to 154 mg/day of clomipramine in inpatients with endogenous depression. The third study contrasted moclobemide to imipramine in DSM-III major depression without endogenous features. "Good responders," according to the CGI for the three studies, were quite similar: for moclobemide, 69.6%, 65.5%, and 57.7%, respectively; and for the TCAs, 70.4%, 71.6%, and 58.4%, respectively. It should be noted, however, that these studies conducted in Brazil and France used a lower dose of TCAs than is typically used in the United States. If higher TCA doses had been used in these studies, the TCAs could possibly have shown a significantly better response than moclobemide.

Angst and Stabl (1992) conducted a meta-analysis of response to moclobemide from the results of response to 1,987 patients who received moclobemide during double-blind comparison trials in which response to other antidepressants (i.e., imipramine, clomipramine, desipramine, amitriptyline, and *second generation* drug types) was compared with moclobemide response. By possible depressive subtypes, the proportions of patients receiving a good/very good CGI rating were as follows: similar results were obtained both for unipolar versus bipolar depression (66% versus 60%, respectively) and for melancholic versus nonmelancholic depression (60% versus 63%, respectively), but the response was slightly greater for agitated than for retarded depression (76% versus 61%, respectively) and for nonpsychotic over psychotic depression (61% versus 54%, respectively). No differences were found between patients who were 65 years of age or younger versus patients who were older than age 65 (65% versus 62%, respectively).

Few studies have focused on the use of moclobemide in atypical versus typical subtypes of depression. Compared with diazepam (a benzodiazepine), moclobemide at 150–450 mg/day was found to be either equivalent (Schweitzer et al. 1989) or worse (Tiller et al. 1989). Larsen and colleagues (1991) contrasted response to moclobemide with responses to isocarboxazid and clomipramine in atypical and typical subtypes with the following protocol: 167 patients were assigned to either 300 mg/day of moclobemide, 30 mg/day of isocarboxazide, or 150 mg/day of clomipramine for a 6-week trial. Generally, the overall differences in response were minimal. The highest response levels were found with moclobemide, followed by isocarboxazide and clomipramine. There was no difference in response between typical and atypical depression patients. Because this trial used only minimal doses of the three antidepressants, it is possible that if the protocol had used dosages closer to maximum (i.e., clomipramine to 300 mg/day and moclobemide to 600 mg/day), the differences in response might have been more pronounced.

Case 2: Bipolar depression.   A 40-year-old woman had a long history of a lack of response to various antidepressants, including TCAs, selective serotonin reuptake inhibitors, and bupropion. Her history included mostly recurrent depression, but there were also brief episodes of hypomania. She reported a 2-month history of progressively worsening major depression. Most recently, she had undergone treatment with up to 80 mg/day of fluoxetine without any long-lasting effects. Before receiving moclobemide, her BDI score was 31, including significant levels of pessimism, thoughts of suicide, irritability, social anhedonia, lack of motivation, insomnia, and lethargy. She was hyperphagic and had rejection hypersensitivity and leaden paralysis, although she had insomnia (late type), not hypersomnia. Her mornings were particularly dysphoric, but she experienced some relief toward evening.

She obtained moclobemide from outside the United States, and within 4 weeks, her BDI score had fallen by 50% to 16, with particular improvement in dysphoria, pessimism, thoughts of suicide, motivation, social anhedonia, and fatigue. She noted improvement even after the initial dose of 150 mg/day; however, there was no change in her level of irritability. With a gradual increase of the dosage to 600 mg/day, the patient maintained improvement; her BDI score fell to as low as 6 after 8 months. Thus, moclobemide may be effective in patients with a background of bipolar disorder that includes symptoms of "typical" depression.

Other Psychiatric Syndromes

Table 2–1 summarizes the clinical response predictors of MAOIs. MAOIs are used for treating problems other than depression (e.g., panic disorder). When major depression coexists with these disorders, it makes sense to consider them as possible treatments. One summary of such applications was completed by Liebowitz and colleagues (1990).

Six studies have reported on the use of MAOIs in panic disorder and agoraphobia. In the treatment and prevention of panic attacks, the effective dose of an MAOI that is equivalent to the efficacy of 150 mg/day of imipramine has been as little as 45 mg/day of phenelzine.

Because rejection hypersensitivity can be part of the definition of atypical depression (and appears to relate to a particularly good response to MAOIs), it is not surprising that social phobia is also a good predictor of response to MAOIs. One study indicated that the percentage of patients who were at least "much improved" was significantly higher in phenelzine patients (64%) than in those receiving either atenolol (30%) or placebo (23%)

Table 2–1. Clinical predictors of response to MAOIs

Clinical parameter	Standard MAOIs	Moclobemide
Bipolar depression	+	+
Atypical depression	+	−
Endogenous depression	±	+
TCA nonresponders	+	?
Panic and depression	+	?

Note. MAOI = monoamine oxidase inhibitor; TCA = tricyclic antidepressant.

(Liebowitz et al. 1990). Further analysis of these data indicated that there was a true advantage of phenelzine over atenolol, especially in the generalized form of social phobia, which is "most likely to be high in interpersonal sensitivity." In social phobia marked by performance anxiety, phenelzine and atenolol appeared similarly effective. One comparative trial of phenelzine and moclobemide showed that both were superior to placebo. Initially, phenelzine appeared to be more effective than moclobemide, but the two response rates evened out by week 16.

Phenelzine has proved to be useful in the treatment of bulimia, with a reduction of binge frequency in 64% of patients, unrelated to the presence of baseline depression. Unfortunately, however, one trial showed that approximately 25% of patients could not tolerate the minimum dosage of 60 mg/day for even 2 weeks.

In patients with borderline personality disorder, tranylcypromine in doses of up to 60 mg/day was helpful primarily for depressive symptoms, and secondarily for antidyscontrol effects. Tranylcypromine was found to be slightly less effective than carbamazepine but more effective than either alprazolam or trifluoperazine.

In open trials and case reports of posttraumatic stress disorder (PTSD), phenelzine has been found to be effective in as many as 73% of patients. In one controlled trial, both phenelzine and imipramine were superior to placebo. Phenelzine was more effective in reducing nightmares and flashbacks than in helping emotional numbness and suppression of war memories, but this result was unrelated to the presence of depression; approximately 25% of patients did not complete the trial because of their reluctance to take medication or because of the onset of side effects.

Biochemical Predictors of Response to MAOIs

Dexamethasone Suppression Test

It had originally been proposed that nonsuppression of plasma cortisol levels or early recovery from the artificial suppression of plasma cortisol levels the day after administration of 1 mg of dexamethasone between 11 P.M. and 12 A.M. might predict a better response to antidepressants (Ribeiro et al. 1993). Most of these studies were conducted with TCAs, however. Usually, patients taking MAOIs and patients taking TCAs were evaluated as one group. Gitlin and colleagues (1984) included 14 patients who were taking a variety of MAOIs in a total of 173 patients who did not have a response associated with pretreatment dexamethasone suppression test (DST) results. In contrast, Coppen and colleagues (1985) included five patients receiving 30 mg of tranylcypromine in a group of 86 patients who were receiving antidepressants. He found that patients with a baseline plasma cortisol of 100 ng/ml or more (nonsuppression) also responded better to antidepressants than those below this cutoff. This was not true for patients whose plasma cortisol levels were above or below the standard post-DST marker level of 50 ng/ml.

The first report to look at the DST with particular relevance to MAOIs came in 1986 when Georgotas et al. reported results of MAOI treatment of 72 outpatients age 55 and older with RDC major depressive disorder (Georgotas et al. 1986). These patients also had a baseline HDRS score of at least 16. Phenelzine was administered in a double-blind procedure at a sufficient dose to keep platelet MAO inhibition above 70%. Patients who responded to treatment were defined as those who no longer met the criteria for major depression and had an HDRS score below 10. By this definition, 14 (58%) phenelzine patients responded. There was no difference in response rate between groups of patients having baseline plasma cortisol levels of 50% ($n = 3$; nonsuppressors) and 61%, ($n = 11$; suppressors).

In a reversal of the original concept, Janicak and colleagues (1987) suggested DST results showing suppressed plasma cortisol might indeed predict a better response to MAOIs. This hypothesis was proposed because nonsuppression of plasma cortisol was associated with melancholia, and positive MAOI response was frequently associated with nonmelancholic atypical depression.

Twenty inpatients who met RDC and DSM-III criteria for major depression were administered up to a maximum of 90 mg/day of phenelzine for a 4-week trial. Patients who responded showed at least a 40% drop in HDRS score; patients who had a partial response showed consistent improvement but did not reach a 40% drop. The results showed that of 9 patients with positive baseline DST results, 7 responded (78%), and 1 (11%) responded partially. In contrast, of 11 patients with negative baseline DST results, only 3 responded (27%), and 1 (9%) responded partially. Similarly, Davidson and colleagues (1988) reported that in 36 depressed inpatients who were administered isocarboxazid, 21 of 24 (88%) patients with positive DST results responded, but only 4 of 12 (33%) with negative DST results responded. Thus, there is some evidence that plasma cortisol suppression may be associated with a better response to MAOIs.

Platelet MAO Activity

Platelet MAO inhibition associated with MAOI treatment has been linked to clinical response. For example, it was shown that in adults in general (Robinson et al. 1978) and in the geriatric population specifically (Georgotas et al. 1981), 80% suppression of baseline platelet MAO activity was associated with a clinical response.

The Robinson et al. report showed a differential response of 68% versus 44% in 62 depressed outpatients. The study by Georgotas et al. contrasted seven of nine patients (78%) who responded to therapy when MAO platelet inhibition was greater than 80% and only one of six (17%) responded when inhibition was less than 80%. Unfortunately, these results do not aid the clinician in choosing an antidepressant.

Baseline platelet MAO activity may be of more use to the clinician; Giller and colleagues (1984) initially reported that patients who responded to isocarboxazid therapy had higher platelet MAO activity than patients who did not respond. A further study of Georgotas and colleagues (1987) is of even greater value in evaluating pretreatment platelet MAO activity. Thirty-seven patients with RDC major depression and a HDRS score of 16 were administered nortriptyline, phenelzine, or placebo. The nortriptyline was adjusted to produce a blood level between 50 and 170 ng/ml; the phenelzine, to produce platelet MAO inhibition of greater than 70% for at least 2 weeks. The negative correlation found between baseline MAO activity and final HDRS score was statistically significant ($r = -.24$, $P < .05$). Twenty-three patients (62%) responded to MAOI therapy and had significantly higher baseline MAO activity (mean = 46.93) than patients who did not respond to MAOI therapy (mean = 30.91, $P < .02$). A review of the published data indicates that a uniformly positive result was found in patients with baseline platelet MAO activity of greater than 50 nmol product/hr/mg protein. There was no difference in the relationship of platelet MAO to response in the nortriptyline or phenelzine groups. Unfortunately, in a further trial by Bresnahan and colleagues (1990), this result was not replicated. The sample consisted of 52 patients who met DSM-III and RDC criteria for "various" depressive disorders. They all received 30–90 mg/day of phenelzine for 4 weeks. Response was defined as a drop of 40% in the baseline HDRS score; partial response was defined as consistent improvement without a 40% drop in baseline HDRS score. Baseline platelet MAO was similar in patients who responded (32.9) and patients who did not respond (28.3). It is possible that results might have been affected by the fact that nine of the 52 patients (17%) did not have unipolar major depression; although only slightly different, the levels of platelet MAO in patients who responded were still greater than in patients who did not respond. Perhaps the clinician can use only the higher levels of platelet MAO as a predictor in unipolar major depression.

Other Biological Measures

Two other possible markers have been investigated in terms of predicting response of MAOIs: cerebral laterality and plasma amino acid profiles. A study by Bruder and colleagues (1990)

Table 2–2. Biological and pharmacological predictors of response to MAOIs

Biological measure	Standard MAOIs	Moclobemide
Dexamethasone suppression test	Suppressors respond better	?
Platelet MAO activity	Baseline > 50 nmol prod/hr/mg protein may respond better	?
Cerebral laterality	—	?
Plasma amino acids	?	—

Note. MAOI = monoamine oxidase inhibitor.

showed that, although cerebral laterality (as determined by dichotic and visual tasks) differentiated patients who would respond to TCA therapy, it did not indicate patients who would respond to MAOI therapy (treatment time = 6 weeks). Similarly, although plasma amino acid concentrations have been useful in predicting response to TCAs, they were not associated with response in 26 patients meeting DSM-III criteria for major depression who were treated with a maximum of 400 mg/day of moclobemide for up to 4 weeks (Moller et al. 1993). Table 2–2 lists a summary of the biochemical predictors of response to MAOIs.

References

Angst J, Stabl M: The efficacy of moclobemide in different patient groups: a meta-analysis of studies. Psychopharmacology 106(suppl):S109–S113, 1992

Biziere K, Berger M: Efficacy of a reversible monoamine oxidase-A inhibitor versus imipramine in subgroups of depressed patients. Acta Psychiatr Scand Suppl 360:59–60, 1990

Bresnahan DB, Pandey GN, Janicak PG, et al: MAO inhibition and clinical response in depressed patients treated with phenelzine. J Clin Psychiatry 51:47–50, 1990

Bruder GE, Stewart JW, Voglmaier MM, et al: Cerebral laterality and depression: relations of perceptual asymmetry to outcome of treatment with tricyclic antidepressants. Neuropsychopharmacology 3:1–10, 1990

Coppen A, Millon P, Harwood J, et al: Does the dexamethasone suppression test predict antidepressant treatment success? Br J Psychiatry 146:294–296, 1985

Davidson JRT, Miller RD, Turnbull CD, et al: Atypical depression. Arch Gen Psychiatry 39:527–534, 1982

Davidson J, Lipper S, Pelton S, et al: The response of depressed inpatients to isocarboxazid. J Clin Psychopharmacol 8:100–107, 1988

Da Prada M, Kettler R, Burkard WP, et al: Some basic aspects of monoamine oxidase-A. Acta Psychiatr Scand Suppl 360:7–12, 1990

Georgotas A, Mann J, Friedman E: Platelet monoamine oxidase inhibition as a potential indicator of favorable response to MAOIs in geriatric depression. Biol Psychiatry 16:997–1001, 1981

Georgotas A, Stokes P, McCue BE, et al: The usefulness of DST in predicting response to antidepressants: a placebo-controlled study. J Affect Disord 11:21–28, 1986

Georgotas A, McCue RE, Friedman E, et al: Prediction of response to nortriptyline and phenelzine by platelet MAO activity. Am J Psychiatry 144:338–340, 1987

Giller E Jr, Bialos D, Harkness L, et al: Assessing treatment response with isocarboxazid. J Clin Psychiatry 45:44–48, 1984

Gitlin NJ, Gwirtsman H, Fairbanks L, et al: Dexamethasone suppression and treatment response. J Clin Psychiatry 45:387–389, 1984

Himmelhoch JM, Detre T, Kupfer DJ, et al: Treatment of previously intractable depressions with tranylcypromine and lithium. J Nerv Ment Dis 155:216–220, 1972

Himmelhoch JM, Fuchs CZ, Symons BJ: A double-blind study of tranylcypromine treatment of major anergic depression. J Nerv Ment Dis 170:628–634, 1982

Himmelhoch JM, Inase NE, Nailinger AG: Tranylcypromine versus imipramine in anergic bipolar depression. Am J Psychiatry 148:910–915, 1991

Janicak PG, Pandey GN, Sharma R, et al: Pretreatment dexamethasone suppression test as a predictor of response to phenelzine. J Clin Psychiatry 48:480–482, 1987

Larsen JK, Gjerris A, Holm P, et al: Moclobemide in depression: a randomized, multicenter trial against isocarboxazide and clomipramine emphasizing atypical depression. Acta Psychiatr Scand 84:564–570, 1991

Lecrubier Y, Guelfi JD: Efficacy of reversible inhibitors of monoamine oxidase-A in various forms of depression. Acta Psychiatr Scand Suppl 360:18–23, 1990

Liebowitz MR, Quitkin FM, Stewart JW, et al: Antidepressant specificity in atypical depression. Arch Gen Psychiatry 45:129–138, 1988

Liebowitz MR, Hollander E, Schneier F, et al: Reversible and irreversible monoamine oxidase inhibitors in other psychiatric disorders. Acta Psychiatr Scand Suppl 360:29–34, 1990

McGrath PJ, Stewart JW, Harrison W, et al: Treatment of tricyclic refractory depression with a monoamine oxidase inhibitor. Psychopharmacol Bull 23:169–172, 1987

McGrath PJ, Stewart JW, Harrison WM, et al: Predictive value of symptoms of atypical depression for differential drug treatment outcome. J Clin Psychopharmacol 12:197–202, 1992

McGrath PJ, Stewart JW, Nunes EV, et al: A double-blind crossover trial of imipramine and phenelzine for outpatients with treatment-refractory depression. Am J Psychiatry 150:118–123, 1993

Moller SE, Danish University Antidepressant Group: Plasma amino acid profiles in relation to clinical response to moclobemide in patients with major depression. J Affect Disord 27:225–231, 1993

Nolen WA, van de Putte JJ, Dijken WA, et al: Treatment strategy in depression. Acta Psychiatr Scand 78:676–683, 1988

Quitkin F, Ritkin A, Klein DF: Monoamine oxidase inhibitors: a review of antidepressant effectiveness. Arch Gen Psychiatry 36:749–760, 1979

Quitkin FM, Stewart JW, McGrath P, et al: Phenelzine versus imipramine in probable atypical depression: defining syndrome boundaries of selective MAO responders. Am J Psychiatry 145:306–311, 1988

Quitkin FM, McGrath PJ, Stewart JW, et al: Phenelzine and imipramine in mood reactive depressives. Arch Gen Psychiatry 46:787–793, 1989

Quitkin FM, McGrath PJ, Stewart JW, et al: Atypical depression, panic attacks, and response to imipramine and phenelzine. Arch Gen Psychiatry 47:935–941, 1990

Ribeiro SCM, Tandon R, Grunhaus L, et al: The DST as a predictor of outcome in depression: a meta-analysis. Am J Psychiatry 150:1618–1629, 1993

Robinson DS, Nies A, Ravaris CL, et al: Clinical pharmacology of phenelzine. Arch Gen Psychiatry 35:629–635, 1978

Schweitzer I, Tiller J, Maguire K, et al: Treatment of atypical depression with moclobemide: a sequential double controlled study. Int J Clin Pharmacol Res IX:111–117, 1989

Spitzer RL, Endicott J, Robins E: Research Diagnostic Criteria: rationale and reliability. Arch Gen Psychiatry 35:773–782, 1978

Stewart JW, McGrath PJ, Quitkin FM, et al: Relevance of DSM-III depressive subtype and chronicity of antidepressant efficacy in atypical depression. Arch Gen Psychiatry 46:1080–1087, 1989

Thase ME, Carpenter K, Kupfer DJ, et al: Clinical significance of reversed vegetative subtypes of recurrent major depression. Psychopharmcol Bull 27:17–22, 1991

Thase ME, Frank E, Mallinger AG, et al: Treatment of imipramine-resistant recurrent depression, III: efficacy of monoamine oxidase inhibitors. J Clin Psychiatry 53:5–11, 1992a

Thase ME, Mallinger AG, McKnight D, et al: Treatment of imipramine-resistant recurrent depression, IV: a double-blind crossover study of tranylcypromine for anergic bipolar depression. Am J Psychiatry 149:195–198, 1992b

Tiller J, Schweitzer I, Maguire K, et al: A sequential double-blind controlled study of moclobemide and diazepam in patients with atypical depression. J Affect Disord 16:181–187, 1989

Versiani M, Oggero U, Atterwain P, et al: A double-blind comparative trial of moclobemide versus imipramine and placebo in major depressive episodes. Br J Psychiatry 155(suppl 6): 72–77, 1989

Versiani M, Nardi AE, Figueira ILV, et al: Tolerability of moclobemide, a new reversible inhibitor of monoamine oxidase-A, compared with other antidepressants and placebo. Acta Psychiatr Scand Suppl 360:24–28, 1990

CHAPTER 3

Newer Antidepressants

Paul J. Goodnick, M.D.

Since the introduction of the tricyclic antidepressants (TCAs) and the monoamine oxidase inhibitors (MAOIs), a series of other types of antidepressants has been introduced in the United States. In 1980, trazodone (triazolopyridine), maprotiline (tetracyclic), and amoxapine (dibenzoxapine TCA metabolite of loxapine) were introduced. These were followed in turn by the development of an entire new class of antidepressants, the selective serotonin reuptake inhibitors (SSRIs), which are the main focus of this chapter. These include (with year of introduction) fluoxetine (1988), sertraline (1992), paroxetine (1993), and fluvoxamine (1994). The unique aminoketone, bupropion, was introduced in 1989; this medication, in contrast to SSRIs, has unique dopaminergic reuptake blockade properties in association with its effects on norepinephrine. In the coming year, two new antidepressants will be released. These are venlafaxine, a phenethylamine with effects on both catecholamines and serotonin, and nefazodone, another triazolopyridine with fewer side effects than trazodone.

In this chapter we focus primarily on known findings regarding SSRIs and bupropion. In this context we demonstrate that clinical and biological information may be quite useful in considering the initial choice of an antidepressant. Such information includes subtype of depression, particular symptoms of depression, and associated symptoms (e.g., obsession-compulsion). Meaningful biological data include baseline serotonin and catecholamine function.

Biological Predictors of Response

The Dexamethasone Suppression Test

The dexamethasone suppression test (DST), as standardized in Carroll and colleagues (1981), is based on one or multiple plasma samples collected at 8 A.M., 4 P.M., and 12 A.M. after administration of 1 mg of dexamethasone at 11 P.M. or 12 A.M. the previous night. A plasma cortisol level of greater than 5 µg/dl is generally considered to be a positive test of nonsuppression. This result has been thought to have a 40%–50% sensitivity and 70%–90% specificity for major depressive disorder (American Psychiatric Association Task Force on Laboratory Tests in Psychiatry 1987). Whereas the earliest studies focused on the DST results as a diagnostic marker, later ones looked at changes in the DST results over the course of treatment. Pooled results have shown that 506 of 699 (72.4%) patients who did not have suppressed cortisol levels at baseline normalized by the time of discharge (Ribeiro et al. 1993). More recently, the DST research focused on the use of the baseline DST results as a predictor of response and long-term outcome, and the use of the posttreatment DST results as a predictor of outcome.

A close evaluation of available research on baseline DST results and response to treatment reveals only three studies that are relevant to newer antidepressants. The first of these examined both maprotiline and trazodone (Simon et al. 1987); the second, sertraline (Peselow et al. 1986); and the third, paroxetine (Peselow et al. 1989). Simon and colleagues reported results of a prospective open study of 34 consecutively admitted inpatients who met DSM-III criteria for major depression. Mean overall age was 39.4 years. There were 12 men and 22 women. Treatment was randomly assigned with patients receiving a mean of 193 mg of maprotiline for 3–7 weeks or 328 mg of trazodone for 3–12 weeks. The dose of each medication was increased "as tolerated, until clinical benefit was evident." Assessment instruments were the Carroll Rating Scale for depression (CRS) and the 17-item Hamilton Depression Rating Scale (HDRS). A positive DST result was determined by a serum cortisol level of greater than 5 µg/dl at 4 P.M. or 11 P.M.; 44% of patients had positive DST results (41% of maprotiline patients and 47% of trazodone patients). Response was defined as "resolution of DSM-III target symptoms" on a five-point global scale. A global rating of fair or poor was considered to be indicative of no response. The authors reported a good to excellent response in 13 of 17 patients in each treatment group. Although the percentage of patients in each group who responded to each medication was greater in groups of patients who did not have suppressed cortisol plasma levels than in groups who did (maprotiline, 86% versus 70%, respectively; trazodone, 88% versus 67%, respectively), these results were not statistically significant. Unfortunately, CRS or HDRS scores were not available to compare changes by DST subgroup. Considering the relatively low number of patients, a Type II error (in which a significant result that would have been found with increased sample size is hidden) might have occurred. Further, a relationship of baseline DST results to final results might have been more evident had dosages been under more strict control.

This study is complemented by a report of inpatients at the New York Veterans Administration Medical Center (Peselow et al. 1986). Patients in the study group met DSM-III criteria for depression and had a minimum score of 18 on the 21-item HDRS. A positive DST result was defined as a plasma cortisol level equal to or greater than 5 µg/ml at 8 A.M., 4 P.M., or 11 P.M. The double-blind protocol included a sertraline dosage of 50–400 mg/day for 4 weeks and a placebo. Unfortunately, this report combined findings on the 16 patients receiving sertraline with 14 others receiving oxaprotiline. Response to treatment was defined as a reduction of at least 50% in the HDRS score and Beck Depression Inventory (BDI) score. Overall, patients with negative DST results had significantly less reduction in HDRS scores ($P < .01$) and BDI scores ($P < .005$) than patients with positive DST results; however, four of five patients with positive DST results responded to sertraline versus five of nine with negative DST results. Similar to the previous report, the authors found within a body of negative results a small sample that had predictable response to sertraline: 80% of patients with positive DST results responded, compared with only 56% of patients with negative DST results. Again, both larger sample size and increased availability of detailed data on this subgroup would have been more useful. As before, the total sample size of 14 patients leads to the possibility of a Type II error.

Finally, a similar lack of response has been reported on DST results and response to paroxetine (Peselow et al. 1989). Criteria for inclusion in this study included a DSM-III diagnosis of depression and a minimum score of 18 on the first 17 items of the HDRS. In this protocol, patients were administered 10–50 mg/day of paroxetine for 6 weeks in a double-blind protocol comparing both imipramine and placebo. A positive DST result was defined as serum cortisol greater than or equal to 5 µg/dl at an 8 A.M. or 4 P.M.. Patients who responded were again defined as having a reduction of at least 50% in HDRS and BDI scores. The 34 paroxetine patients included 21 men and 13 women with a mean age of 44.3 years. In this paroxetine group, 17 of 34 patients responded, and the rate of response in groups with both positive and negative DST results was identical (6 of 12 and 11 of 22, respectively, both 50%). Thus, in these three studies relating baseline DST results to medication response, results that contrasted the percentage of patients who responded to medication with the percentage of patients who did not respond indicated no significant differences; however, taking the small sample sizes into consideration, a significant differential may exist for those medications that show the greatest difference between percentages of patients with positive versus negative DST results. For example, sertraline ($\delta = 24\%$) and trazodone ($\delta = 21\%$) may be favored over maprotiline ($\delta = 16\%$) and paroxetine ($\delta = 0\%$).

Measures of Neurochemical Function as Predictors

Serotonergic and catecholaminergic function are thought to be relevant to predicting response based on current theories of depression and of the method of antidepressant action. Older theories of depression have been based on low levels of synaptic serotonin, norepinephrine, or dopamine. More recent theories are based upon supersensitive postsynaptic serotonergic and catecholaminergic receptors. Furthermore, many more recent antidepressants appear to be more specific in their effects on biochemical amines: the tetracyclic maprotiline is noradrenergic; trazodone is a postsynaptic 5-hydroxytryptamine (5-HT) agonist; the SSRIs (fluoxetine, sertraline, paroxetine, fluvoxamine) are as named, selective serotonin reuptake inhibitors; and bupropion is a reuptake blocker/agonist of dopamine and norepinephrine. For these reasons, it is quite logical to expect a relationship to exist between some baseline neurochemical values and antidepressant response.

For serotonergic antidepressants, the most logical measures are those of platelet function, plasma reuptake, concentration ratios of tryptophan in plasma, levels of cerebrospinal metabolites, and neuroendocrine responses to serotonergic agents. There have been seven reports on peripheral blood measures of serotonin and antidepressant response.

The earliest report merely related that platelet-rich plasma 5-HT concentrations dropped by 95% ($P < .001$) during the successful treatment of obsessive-compulsive disorder and depression with fluoxetine (Pigott et al. 1990). The next study, although finding significant impact of fluvoxamine on the reuptake inhibition of 5-HT, did not include data regarding any possible relationship of baseline 5-HT measures to therapeutic response (Nathan et al. 1990). Similarly, studies in normal volunteers showed that fluvoxamine treatment significantly reduced whole blood 5-HT concentration (Kremer et al. 1990).

The first attempt to relate therapeutic outcome of SSRIs to baseline measures of 5-HT came one year later (Muck-Seler et al. 1991). Included in a total of 48 inpatients meeting Research Diagnostic Criteria (RDC) for unipolar major depression (Spitzer et al. 1978) were 25 men and 23 women with a mean age of 45.5 years. Medications were given to a selected number of patients as follows: clovoxamine, 13; trazodone, 12; amitriptyline, 10; maprotiline, 8; fluvoxamine, 5. Response was defined as a decrease in HDRS scores of 50% or more. Statistical consideration of the relationship between posttreatment platelet 5-HT and final outcome was studied by correlation coefficient, but its value ($r = .02$) was not significant. There was no attempt to relate baseline 5-HT to change in HDRS score. Also, no data were provided on treatment response to trazodone. Further, the mixed reuptake inhibitor amitriptyline was combined with the SSRIs clovoxamine and fluvoxamine to evaluate response to "serotonergic" antidepressants. It is well known that amitriptyline has, at best, a balance of effects on 5-HT and on catecholamines. The sample size was too small to look at baseline 5-HT differences between patients who responded ($n = 3$) and patients who did not respond ($n = 2$) to fluvoxamine. Thus, in terms of testing the predictability of

5-HT measures to determine SSRI response, this study is of little assistance.

The next study examined response after 6 weeks of treatment of 100 mg/day of fluvoxamine (Celada et al. 1992). This was given to 11 patients who met the DSM-III-R criteria for major depressive disorder and had an HDRS score of 17 or more. Patients included 7 women and 4 men with a mean age of 42.5 years. Platelet 5-HT was determined by platelet counting in order to obtain total serotonin per platelet. Results showed that patients with an HDRS score under 10 after 6 weeks had pretreatment platelet 5-HT concentrations significantly lower than those who improved later (516 versus 840 ng/10^9 platelets, $P < .02$). This study is limited by a small sample size and subtherapeutic doses (100 mg/day) and blood levels (mean of 60 ng/ml) of fluvoxamine. The standard doses and therapeutic blood level ranges for fluvoxamine are 100–300 mg/day and 160–220 ng/ml, respectively (Goodnick 1994).

Another prospective study examined the response of 46 patients who met DSM-III-R criteria for major depressive disorder to fluoxetine therapy (Lu et al. 1992). Patients who responded were defined as those with a drop in HDRS score of more than 50%. No differences were found in pretreatment platelet 5-HT between patients who responded (1.15, SD = .53) and patients who did not respond (1.38, SD = .55). A recent report by Tollefson, presented at the 1994 American Psychiatric Association meeting in Philadelphia, showed that higher baseline values of platelet K_d [^{3}H]-imipramine were associated with change in HDRS score ($r = .22$, $P = .06$) and response status ($P < .05$) in patients receiving imipramine or fluoxetine on a double-blind basis.

The author has preliminary results from two open-label studies of sertraline and paroxetine. In each study, patients who met DSM-III-R criteria for major depressive disorder were included. In the paroxetine study, 14 patients were treated with 20 mg/day of paroxetine for 8 weeks. Patients who responded with a decrease in HDRS score of at least 50% had a significantly higher baseline platelet 5-HT content (60.7 ± 28.4 ng/10^8 platelets) than patients who did not respond (23.0 ± 29.9 ng/10^8 platelets, $P = .03$). Furthermore, baseline platelet 5-HT correlated significantly with change in BDI score ($r = .77$, $P < .005$) (Goodnick et al. 1995).

In the sertraline study, patients who met DSM-III-R criteria for major depressive disorder were treated with 50 mg/day for

8 weeks. In nine patients who completed therapy, a significant correlation was found between higher baseline platelet 5-HT content (mean = 70.5, SD = 16.5 ng/10^8 platelets) and change in BDI score (r = .67, P < .05). The baseline platelet serotonin content did not predict change in HDRS score because of the relatively uniform significant response to sertraline (21, SD = 5.6).

Another approach has been to look at plasma ratios of tryptophan to neutral amino acids. Plasma tryptophan concentrations have been examined as predictors of response to paroxetine (Moller et al. 1990). In a double-blind protocol, 27 patients who met DSM-III criteria for major depressive disorder received a fixed dose of paroxetine up to a maximum of 30 mg/day for 4 weeks. Eighty-one percent of the patients in the group were women with a mean age of 50 years. During the course of treatment, the mean 17-item HDRS score dropped from 24.1 (SD = 4.9) to 13.1 (SD = 4.2). Lower baseline plasma tryptophan (mean = 35.3 ± 10.1 nmol/ml) was found to be significantly correlated with later paroxetine response as seen in HDRS score improvement (r = ± .40, P < .05).

Yet another study looked at cerebrospinal fluid concentrations as predicting response to 20 mg/day of fluoxetine in nine patients who met RDC and DSM-III-R criteria for a major depressive disorder. Because the baseline levels of 5-hydroxyindoleactic acid (5-HIAA) were slightly but not significantly lower than controls (95.9 versus 111.2 pmol/ml, respectively), no relationship was found between the degree of improvement on fluoxetine and baseline biochemistry (De Bellis et al. 1993). Clinical response to fluoxetine was modest (from 23.2, SD = 6.5 to 17.4, SD = 5.0) on the HDRS score.

Neuroendocrine challenge tests have been used to evaluate serotonergic predictability of response to serotonergic drugs. The earliest reported study of prolactin response to intravenous tryptophan (Price et al. 1989) included 30 patients who met DSM-III-R criteria for major depressive disorder. Of these 30 patients, 28 were unipolar, and 2 were bipolar. Twenty-one of the 28 unipolar patients met DSM-III-R criteria for melancholia; 8 had a mood-congruent psychosis. In the double-blind protocol, fluvoxamine treatment was initiated at a dose of 100 mg and increased to a target of 300 mg/day. Overall, based on a 25-item HDRS, there was only a modest decrease in the HDRS score from 35 (SD = 10) to 28 (SD = 14); by that author's criteria, only eight of the 30 patients showed a positive response. The 4-hour test was performed intravenously after an overnight fast. Plasma prolactin samples were collected by indwelling catheter 15 and .5 minutes before infusion, and 30, 40, 50, 60, 70, and 90 minutes after infusion of tryptophan. While baseline change in area under the curve (dAUC) prolactin correlated positively with baseline HDRS score severity ($r = .37, P < .05$), no relationship was found between fluvoxamine response and either dAUC or peak change in serum prolactin (dPrl). This result could have easily been influenced by the overall lack of clinical response to fluvoxamine.

More recently, prolactin response to 60 mg of the 5-HT releaser, fenfluramine, was investigated (Malone et al. 1993). In 10 patients with DSM-III-R major depression who were treated with various SSRIs, four of five patients who responded to treatment had an increase in plasma prolactin level. In contrast, three of four patients who did not respond showed a decrease in plasma prolactin after treatment. Unfortunately, no details are available regarding medication doses, degree of response to medication, and the possible relationship of baseline prolactin response to fenfluramine and change in depressive response.

A related study on DSM-III-R obsessive-compulsive disorder evaluated the response of 10 patients who received fluoxetine for 8 weeks, with a dose of 40 mg/day for a minimum of 2 weeks (Hollander et al. 1993). In terms of overall therapeutic response and association of the prolactin response with meta-chlorophenylpiperazine (MCPP), this patient group was combined with another that received up to 300 mg/day of clomipramine for up to 10 weeks. The overall mean clinical global improvement (CGI) score was 2.38 ± 1.45. Increased prolactin blunting was correlated with a suboptimal treatment response ($r = .40, P = .06$). When MCPP induced an increase in prolactin of more than 3 ng/ml, 7 of 7 patients responded; only 5 of 9 responded when it was less than 3 ng/ml.

A further study has examined prolactin response to thyrotropin-releasing hormone (TRH) as a possible predictor of response to fluoxetine (Rosenbaum et al. 1993). In 33 patients with DSM-III-R major depression, fluoxetine was administered at 20 mg/day for 8 weeks. In the TRH test, patients were given 400 μg iv of TRH after an overnight fast. Plasma samples were taken at baseline and after 10, 20, 30, 45, 60, and 90 minutes to evaluate prolactin levels. The degree of prolactin response at 20, 30, and 45 minutes after the TRH test, as well as the peak change after the TRH test, significantly predicted response (at 20 minutes, $r = .35$, $P < .04$; at 30 minutes, $r = .37$, $P < .04$; at 45 minutes, $r = .35$, $P = .05$; at peak, $r = .35$, $P = .04$). The mean peak changes in prolactin levels were 28.3 ± 17.7 for patients who experienced anger attacks and 52.2 ± 18.4 for patients who did not. Rosenbaum's group explained that this result is related to the hypothesized serotonin inhibition of TRH. Thus, low central serotonergic availability leads to hypersecretion of TRH with secondary desensitization of pituitary cell receptors, and the more exaggerated responses occur because of effects from the lack of 5-HT. Serotonergic medication is in a position to correct this deficiency. The most recent reported results concerning the relationship of fluoxetine response in major depression to serotonergic measures were presented at the 1995 meeting of the American Psychiatric Association (Falk et al. 1995). Thirteen patients meeting DSM-III-R criteria for major depressive disorder were first tested for degree of increase of serum prolactin following administration of 60 mg of the serotonin-releaser, fenfluramine. An increase of less than six is considered a "blunted" response. With blood drawn over a course of 5 hours after PO fenfluramine administration, patients were assigned randomly on a double-blind basis to either fluoxetine 20 mg or placebo for 11 weeks. Among the seven responders (decrease of HDRS of >6), there was a significant negative correlation between peak prolactin response to fenfluramine and time required to first show responses to fluoxetine ($r = .93$, $P < .001$).

It appears, therefore, that indicators of serotonergic hypofunction or hypersensitivity can predict response to serotonergic antidepressants. Neuroendocrine investigations provide the greatest support for this hypothesis (3 of 4, 75%); somewhat less support is provided in studies of platelet function and biochemical concentrations (4 of 7, 57%). Of the three studies that do not support the use of serotenergic activity as a predictor of antidepressant response, factors that influence the possibility of finding a relationship between serotonin variables and response to an SSRI include mixing the types of medications—for example, mixing an SSRI with a TCA (Muck-Seler et al. 1991)—and an overall lack of clinical response to the SSRI (De Bellis et al. 1993; Price et al. 1989). When the SSRI medication type is specified, the rates of finding predictability are 2 of 4 for fluoxetine (50%), 1 of 1 for sertraline (100%), 2 of 2 for paroxetine (100%), and 1 of 3 for fluvoxamine (33%). These results might also be explained by the more positive results found in SSRI medications that are relatively more serotonin-specific (i.e., sertraline and paroxetine) than in medications that are relatively less specific (i.e., fluoxetine and fluvoxamine) (Palmer and Benfield, 1994). If these studies are replicated, those patients who have relatively higher levels of platelet 5-HT content, lower plasma tryptophan, and exaggerated prolactin responses to neuroendocrine challenges with TRH, fenfluramine, or MCPP, may be better candidates for antidepressant treatment with the most specific SSRIs, sertraline and paroxetine.

Case 1: Major depression with low 5-HT.   A 51-year-old white woman presented with a 4-month history of worsening thoughts of death, low concentration, low energy, and anhedonia. Her symptoms were exacerbated by problems with her husband, making her too depressed to handle even a part-time job. She met DSM-III-R criteria for major depression and had a BDI score of 32 and an HDRS score of 18. She had previously not responded to the catecholaminergic medication, bupropion. Her platelet 5-HT content exceeded 80 ng/10^8. She was administered 20 mg of paroxetine per day and showed significant improvement at week 4, manifested by a fall in BDI and HDRS scores to 8 and 5, respectively, which were then maintained. Although she still had marital difficulties, she was able to assert herself and begin full-time employment. The serotonergic-specific medication was successful in biochemically addressing her deficiency.

Case 2: Major depression with diabetes mellitus and low 5-HT.   A 38-year-old woman presented with significant symptoms of dysphoria, anhedonia, insomnia, retardation, fatigue, feelings of worthlessness and guilt, impaired concentration, and thoughts of death; her depressive condition had progressively deteriorated for 2.5 years, and she was diabetic. Her HDRS score was 23, her BDI score was 20, and her baseline platelet 5-HT was approximately 70 ng/10^8. By the end of 2 weeks of treatment with sertraline, her HDRS score had dropped to 8 (more than 67%). By the end of 2 months, not only had her depression improved, but her dietary compliance had jumped significantly from 25% to 70%. She was more sociable, interacted better with others, and was happier and more effective at her job. She had previously not responded to either trazodone or fluoxetine, probably because of trazodone's relative lack of effect on serotonin specificity.

Catecholamine measures have been less frequently studied in the newer medications, but some data do exist for SSRIs and bupropion. Unfortunately, the earliest available study (Schildkraut et al. 1992) reported only that 6 weeks of fluoxetine treatment produced statistically significant decreases in urinary output of norepinephrine and its metabolites. There is no report of any possible association of baseline catecholamine measures and clinical response.

The next report by Salzman and colleagues (1993) included a group of five patients receiving paroxetine (a maximum of 50 mg/day) and another five patients receiving fluoxetine (a maximum of 80 mg/day) for 12 weeks. Baseline and change in measures of plasma homovanillic acid (HVA) were reported. For this combined treatment group, mean baseline HVA did not differentiate between patients responding with a reduction in HDRS score of more than 50% or less than 50%; however, patients who responded showed a mean decrease in HVA, whereas patients who did not respond showed a mean increase. A regression analysis relating percentage change in plasma HVA with percentage change in HDRS score was significant ($r = .70$, $P < .02$). Because paroxetine is more specific to 5-HT than fluoxetine, the lack of baseline predictability might have been affected by combining treatment groups.

Fluvoxamine, with fewer laboratory noradrenergic effects than fluoxetine, was evaluated further in a 6-week multicenter treatment study of 54 outpatients with DSM-III-R major depressive disorder (Johnson et al. 1993). Its efficacy was contrasted to imipramine and placebo. Urine samples were collected for measurement of MHPG, vanillylmandelic acid, metanephrine, and normetanephrine; plasma norepinephrine was also measured. Of the 38 patients who could provide complete urine collections, 12 received a mean of 223 ± 60 mg/day of fluvoxamine. Fifteen patients completed plasma norepinephrine evaluations; their mean fluvoxamine dose was similar to that of the other 12 patients. Clinical response to fluvoxamine was 46% in patients with collected urine samples and 47% in those with collected plasma samples. Although specific data were not reported, no relationship was found between any baseline or change measure of catecholamine function and fluvoxamine response.

Similarly, preliminary results in the author's study of paroxetine (discussed previously) showed that neither baseline levels nor changes in plasma MHPG and HVA could predict response.

Thus, for the SSRIs, there has been no catecholamine measure to date that is useful for predicting antidepressant response. This is not surprising, because the predominant effect, as reflected in the classification's name, is to influence serotonin, not catecholamine function.

Bupropion is an aminoketone antidepressant with specific dopaminergic and noradrenergic effects with no influence on 5-HT parameters (Ferris et al. 1983). Two studies have reported results on the biochemical effects of bupropion and clinical response. The earlier double-blind study examined doses of up to 500 mg/day of bupropion for treatment of depression (Golden et al. 1988). That group did not find baseline measures of plasma HVA related to outcome. Six patients who responded (with a reduction in HDRS score of either 10 points or more or 50% from baseline scores) had an initial plasma HVA of 41.7 ± 4.0 pmol/ml; four patients who did not respond had an initial plasma HVA of 52.1 ± 5.7 pmol/ml. This difference was not statistically significant, but it could have been due to the small sample size. Plasma HVA, however, rose significantly in patients who did not respond to 70.9 ± 5.6 pmol/ml ($P < .02$), but response values, with a final mean level of 42.1 ± 3.3 pmol/ml, did not change. In the second study on treatment of chronic fatigue syndrome (Goodnick et al. 1992), the dose of 300 mg/day of bupropion did not show any relationship between baseline plasma MHPG or HVA and response; however, a decrease in plasma HVA correlated significantly with response ($r = .96, P < .01$). Among the seven patients with available data, the decrease in plasma HVA occurred in all patients who responded with a decrease in HDRS score of at least 40%. In the one of the patients who completed two sets of laboratory tests, plasma HVA increased.

These results, unfortunately, do not help in predicting outcome to bupropion in advance. It is certainly possible that with larger sample populations, both dopaminergic and noradrenergic variables may prove to be related to clinical outcome. Such a study is currently under way by the author, in collaboration with Dr. Charles L. Bowden and Dr. C. Lindsay DeVane. This study examines plasma HVA, plasma MHPG, and a timed 7-hour urine collection to analyze noradrenergic metabolites in a sample of patients receiving 300 mg/day of controlled-release bupropion for 8 weeks.

Table 3–1 summarizes the biochemical predictors of response to the newer antidepressants.

Clinical Predictors of Response to Newer Antidepressants

As described previously, there have been relatively few studies of biological predictors of response to newer antidepressants. Thus, clinical predictors of response must be considered. These include symptoms of major depression and other associated conditions such as panic disorder, generalized anxiety disorder, obsessive-compulsive disorder, and a history of mania or hypomania.

Characteristics of the Depressive Disorder

Fluoxetine. Fluoxetine has been reported (Kasper et al. 1992) to yield better responses in patients with prominent psychomotor retardation than in patients with agitated depression after 2–3 weeks, according to unpublished data from the Lilly Research Center.

Reimherr and colleagues (1984) reported on 110 patients who met criteria for DSM-III major depressive disorder who were given fluoxetine (40–80 mg/day) or imipramine (150–300 mg/day) for 4 weeks. At the end of treatment, patients who responded had "moderate or marked improvement" (considered similar to a decrease in HDRS scores of 50% or more). Factors that appeared to separate patients who responded to fluoxetine from those who responded to imipramine were a past history of lack of response (43% versus 30%, respectively) and a history of greater than 2 years of depressive symptoms with (59% versus 29%, respectively) or without (33% versus 20%, respectively) recent exacerbation. Parameters of agitation and psychomotor retardation were not specifically evaluated.

Table 3–1. Human biochemistry and response to newer antidepressants

Medication class	Medication	DST positive	Serotonin tests	Catecholamine tests
Triazolopyridines	Trazodone	86% vs. 67%	No results	No results
SSRI	Total	1/2 = 50%	6/9 = 67% Plt 5-HT (I) Plt Trp (D) TRH-Pr1 (I)	0/3 = 0%
SSRI	Fluoxetine	No results	3/5 = 60%	No PreRX data on HVA
SSRI	Sertraline	80% > 56%	1/1 = 100%	No results
SSRI	Paroxetine	Negative	2/2 = 100%	0/2 = 0
SSRI	Fluvoxamine	No results	1/3 = 33%	0/1 = 0%
Aminoketone	Bupropion	No results	No results	? trend for higher Plt HVA in nonresponders

Note. DST = dexamethasone suppression test; SSRI = selective serotonin reuptake inhibitor; Plt = platelet; 5-HT = 5-hydroxytryptamine; Trp = tryptophan; TRH = thyrotropin-releasing hormone; TRH-Prl = TRH-induced change in prolactin; I = increased; D = decreased; HVA = homovanillic acid.

Laakmann and colleagues (1988) contrasted 40 mg/day of fluoxetine with 100 mg/day of amitriptyline in a 5-week treatment trial. The 130 patients who participated had a minimum HDRS score of 18 points on the first 17 items; no specific diagnostic criteria were listed. A comparison of response in patients who received flouxetine showed the following mean reductions in HDRS scores by depressive subtypes: 13.6 points for patients with retarded depression, 21.1 points for patients with "vitally disturbed" or endogenous depression, and approximately 15 points for patients with "anxious-agitated" depression. It should be noted that exact data were provided only for the first two groups. Thus, the agitation subtype of depression responded only marginally better than the psychomotor retarded subtype.

Taneri and Kohler (1989) replicated the Lilly Corporation results that indicated that patients with retarded depression had a better response to fluoxetine than patients with agitated depression. In their study of 28 patients who met ICD 300.40 or 298.00 (neurotic or reactive depressive disorder) and had a minimum HDRS score of 17, patients received 40 mg/day of fluoxetine or 150 mg/day of nomifensine. No detailed data on the subgroups were presented.

A detailed report was then published by the Lilly Corporation (Beasley et al. 1991) of 698 patients who met DSM-III criteria for depression and had an HDRS score of 20 or more on the 21-item form. Patients were grouped according to whether they had a baseline presence of agitation ($n = 125$), retardation ($n = 187$), or neither ($n = 386$). This study contrasted the response to up to 60 mg/day of fluoxetine with the response to up to 300 mg/day of imipramine, and the response to placebo. Mean changes in HDRS scores in each of the three groups with at least 4 weeks of fluoxetine therapy were very similar (agitated, 11.3; retarded, 11.1; and neither, 12.4). Scores in each of the three depression types, however, were greater than scores from the placebo group (agitated, 7.9; retarded, 7.8; and neither, 6.9; $P < .05$). Fluoxetine was associated with more activating events (28%) than imipramine (21%) or placebo (17%).

There have been a series of more recent papers on the clinical aspects of fluoxetine response in depression. In a multicenter protocol, Bowden and colleagues (1993) reported results of 58 patients who met DSM-III-R criteria for major depressive disorder who received up to 60 mg of fluoxetine or 250 mg of desipramine on a double-blind randomized basis. Overall, 64% of the fluoxetine and 68% of the desipramine patients were found to have a reduction in HDRS scores of 50% or more during treatment. When patients who were severely ill (HDRS scores of 24 or more) were separated from those who were moderately ill (HDRS scores of less than 24), there was no difference in response between the two drugs; however, among fluoxetine patients, there was a higher response rate (82%, $P = .1$) for patients with less severe anxiety than for the more anxious patients (50%).

In a reevaluation of 3,183 outpatients and inpatients with major depressive disorder (according to RDC) who participated in one of 19 double-blind, randomized clinical trials of fluoxetine versus placebo or TCA, Pande and Sayler (1993) found that there was no difference in the rate of response (as measured by a drop in HDRS score of 50% or more) between mild, moderate, or severely depressed patients (56%, 60%, and 63%, respectively). A follow-up of this same patient base (Tollefson et al. 1994a) found a relatively greater degree of significant response to fluoxetine compared with placebo in the "anxious subgroup" (defined as an anxiety or somatization HDRS factor score—the sum of items 10–13, 15, and 17—of 7 or more). Overall, response to fluoxetine was significant for the anxious group ($P < .001$) and for the nonanxious group ($P = .026$) of patients who responded. The difference between the number of patients who responded in the anxious group versus the nonanxious group was not significant (55.7% versus 60.7%, respectively).

Another study was conducted in which 671 patients at least 60 years old meeting DSM-III-R criteria for unipolar major depressive disorder were studied for response to 20 mg/day of fluoxetine versus placebo in a double-blind protocol (Tollefson and Holman, 1993). Baseline cognitive and psychomotor retardation scores were found to be predictive of response to fluoxetine.

In terms of other subtypes of depressive disorders, publications on dysthymic disorder, "atypical depression," and bipolar disorder can be found. Regarding dysthymia, one recent study of 20 patients meeting DSM-III-R criteria attempted to contrast the response of patients who were given either 20–60 mg/day of fluoxetine with patients who received 50–350 mg/day of trazodone (Rosenthal et al. 1992). This open-label study had follow-ups

3 and 5 months after the initiation of therapy. At 3 months, 8 of 11 fluoxetine patients (72.7%) and 4 of 6 trazodone patients (66.7%) showed a reduction in HDRS score of over 50% from a mean baseline of 13.8. At 3 months, this improvement was maintained by only four of 11 fluoxetine patients (36.4%) and 3 of 6 trazodone patients (50%).

There are two studies (Goodnick and Extein 1989; Stratta et al. 1991) that influence the use of fluoxetine in patients with atypical depression. These patients have depressive symptoms that are characterized by hyperphagia and hypersomnia, as well as lack of mood response and increased sensitivity to rejection. The initial open DSM-III-R trial compared 23 patients receiving 40 mg/day of fluoxetine with 34 patients receiving 450 mg/day of bupropion for 8 weeks (Goodnick and Extein 1989). Among the fluoxetine patients, 13 were "typical" (i.e., with insomnia and anorexia), 9 were atypical (with hypersomnia and hyperphagia), and 1 had bipolar characteristics. A significant response to fluoxetine was seen in typical depression (mean drop in BDI score was 11.8, $P < .003$), but not in atypical depression (mean drop in BDI score was 3.1, $P = $ NS). The proportion of patients with improvement in BDI scores of more that 50% was 7 of 13 (54%) for patients with typical depression and 2 of 9 (22%) for patients with atypical depression.

In the second study, 28 patients who met the criteria described in a report by Quitkin and colleagues (1988) for atypical depression were administered either 20 mg/day of fluoxetine or a maximum of 75 mg/day of imipramine for 5 weeks (Stratta et al. 1991). Overall, both medications were equally effective in producing a mean reduction in HDRS scores of 8 for fluoxetine and 8.8 for imipramine. Patients receiving fluoxetine, however, reached significant improvement in HDRS scores sooner than those receiving imipramine (day 14 versus day 21) and showed better results in certain measures from the Atypical Depressive Disorders Scale (change in sleep, limb heaviness, and social difficulties). Unfortunately, this study is biased in favor of fluoxetine because of the 75 mg subtherapeutic dose of imipramine used (the standard dose is 150–300 mg). A recent, large open study indicated that fluoxetine may be beneficial in atypical depression (F. Quitkin, personal communication, June, 1994).

In bipolar II depression (i.e., major depression with a background of hypomania), fluoxetine was shown to be effective relatively early (Goodnick and Extein 1989). Two studies have been conducted since that time (Cohn et al. 1989; Simpson and Depaulo, 1991).

The first study included 89 patients who met the following criteria: 1) DSM-III criteria for "bipolar disorder"; 2) a minimum score of 20 on the 21-item HDRS; and 3) at least one "distinct manic episode" in the previous 5 years. Over a period of 6 weeks, patients received either a maximum of 80 mg/day of fluoxetine or 300 mg/day of imipramine. Patients who responded were defined as those who showed an improvement in HDRS scores of 50% or more. Unfortunately, only 57% of fluoxetine and 47% of imipramine patients completed the 6-week trial. Overall, mean HDRS score improved by 13.9 in fluoxetine patients and 9.7 in imipramine patients. For patients completing at least 3 weeks of therapy, the response rate was 18 of 21 (86%) for fluoxetine, 12 of 21 (57%) for imipramine, and 5 of 8 (38%) for placebo. In the second report, 13 patients who met RDC for bipolar II disorder received an open trial of 20–60 mg/day of fluoxetine. Ten of the 13 (77%) who had not responded previously achieved a good or very good response after taking fluoxetine for 10 or more months.

Also important are those factors that may be predictors of either a poor response to fluoxetine or of complications from its use. One report (Cain 1992) stated that nonresponse may be due to a "therapeutic window" effect in which standard doses of fluoxetine may actually be too high for some depressed patients. Also, it has been found that the mean brain:plasma ratio for fluoxetine and its metabolite, norfluoxetine, is 2.6 (Renshaw et al. 1992). Thus, patients who receive too much fluoxetine may experience more toxic effects. Finally, some bipolar patients may be likely to cycle into mania after receiving fluoxetine. Data from Lilly Corporation indicate that the rate of mania in unipolar and bipolar patients receiving fluoxetine was .98%; in those receiving TCAs (which are well known for this complication), the rate of mania was only .39% (Goodnick 1992).

Thus, fluoxetine has been seen at times to be more effective in retarded than in agitated depression, but usually both groups have responded equally well. Furthermore, the usefulness of fluoxetine in atypical depression is significantly limited; the only positive study to this effect was biased by dosage levels in favor of fluoxetine. Fluoxetine may indeed be effective for bipolar depression; however, its risk of inducing mania may be several times that of TCAs. Thus, although it is effective overall in major depression, and in particular, "endogenous" depression, there are few depression-associated predictors of response.

Sertraline. Sertraline has been available in the United States since February 1992. Although generally effective in major depression (Murdoch and McTavish 1992), few studies have examined its effectiveness by possible subtypes of depression. The only study that made a significant contribution in this area is that of Reimherr and colleagues (1990). In this 8-week study, a maximum of 200 mg/day was administered to 135 patients who met DSM-III criteria for major depression in a double-blind comparison with amitriptyline and placebo. Single-episode patients responded (i.e., HDRS scores decreased by 50% or more) slightly more than patients with recurrent episodes (62% versus 52%, respectively), and melancholic patients responded slightly more than nonmelancholic patients (56% versus 50%, respectively), although the differences are relatively minimal. The most recent result reported shows that seasonal affective disorder (SAD) may predict a positive response to sertraline at a dose of up to 200 mg/day. A double-blind random-assignment placebo-controlled multicenter study showed a reduction of 51.8% in SAD items and of 47.6% in HDRS ($P < .05$ both within and between groups) (Moscovitch et al. 1995).

Paroxetine. This medication was released in the United States in February 1993. Virtually all sponsored studies conducted for the purpose of obtaining FDA approval found no symptom or depression subcategory particularly favorable or unfavorable to response. One study attempted to contrast paroxetine to clomipramine in a multicenter trial (Danish University Antidepressant Group 1990). Patients who met DSM-III criteria for depression and who had an HDRS score of at least 18 on the first 17 items were classified by scores on the Newcastle scale as endogenous (greater than 5.5) or nonendogenous (less than 5.5). Patients received a 6-week course of either 30 mg/day of paroxetine or 150 mg/day of clomipramine. From the 2nd week forward, clomipramine was associated with a better response than paroxetine. In addition, at the end of the 6th week, complete response (HDRS score of less than

7) was shown in 50%–60% of clomipramine patients but only 20%–25% of paroxetine patients. These differences, however, could not be explained by earlier manic/depressive ratings, duration of illness, or diagnostic ratings (including endogenicity). Paroxetine was recently found to be efficacious in an open design protocol in a retrospective review of 20 patients who met DSM-III-R criteria for bipolar disorder. These patients had all "failed" treatment with at lease one standard antidepressant agent; a response rate of 65% and a rate of induced mania of 10% were found (Baldassano et al. 1995).

Fluvoxamine.   This medication has recently been released in the United States, and it is already in widespread use in Canada. There have been several attempts to depict particular indicators for future response to fluvoxamine. At the Connecticut Mental Health Center, 38 patients who had previously had no response to TCAs were administered up to 200 mg/day of fluvoxamine for 4–6 weeks (Delgado et al. 1988). Patients who responded were classified as having either a "partial" (if there was an overall improvement that was maintained) or a "marked" (if the HDRS score dropped by more than 50% with a final score of 15 or less) response. Of 28 patients who completed therapy, 8 (29%) responded (3 partial, 5 marked) to fluvoxamine alone. Patients who responded "tended to be older and to have a later age at onset, fewer previous ineffective antidepressant trials, fewer prior episodes, and fewer hospitalizations than non-responders, but these differences were not statistically significant."

Another study (Kasper et al. 1990) including 42 patients with ICD-9 major depression examined changes in HDRS score of greater than 30% in response to total sleep deprivation before and after the administration of 100–300 mg of fluvoxamine. All but one patient met DSM-III criteria for major depression. Neither the day-1 nor the day-2 response to total sleep deprivation was related to the antidepressant treatment.

The only other meaningful results came from a study conducted in Italy (Gasperini et al. 1992). Fifty-six patients who met DSM-III-R criteria for major depression were given a maximum of 150 mg/day of amitriptyline and 300 mg/day of fluvoxamine for up to 6 weeks. Two different criteria were used to identify response: 1) a standard HDRS score reduction of more than 50%, and 2) HDRS scores of less than 17 with residual symptoms not affecting usual social and work activities. Symptoms of anxiety and middle and late insomnia were associated with better fluvoxamine response. Worse response to fluvoxamine was related to higher diurnal mood variation and greater psychomotor retardation.

Thus, clinical information linked to type of depression in the use of fluvoxamine is relatively unavailable. It is interesting, however, that the Gasperini study found psychomotor retardation to be a negative predictor for fluvoxamine, because it had previously been considered a possible positive predictor for fluvoxamine.

Bupropion. This aminoketone has been subject to only a few reports concerning its use with depressive disorder subtypes. Some reports have focused on the use of bupropion in both atypical and cyclical depressions (mostly bipolar).

In a 1989 study, the response to 450 mg/day of bupropion for 8 weeks was contrasted among subtypes of patients who met DSM-III-R criteria for major depression: 9 had bipolar II depression, 14 had atypical depression, and 11 had "typical" insomniac/anorectic depression (Goodnick and Extein 1989); mean changes in the BDI score were 16.3 ($P < .003$), 12.6 ($P < .001$), and 6.0 ($P = .09$), respectively. A significant decrease of less than 50% in BDI scores was found in 8 of 9 (89%) patients with bipolar disorder, 9 of 14 (64%) patients with atypical depression, and only 2 of 11 (18%) patients with typical depression. In a follow-up study of eight bipolar II patients and 15 atypical depression patients, 15 (65%) showed a significant decrease of more than 50% in the BDI score (Goodnick 1992). When the patient group was limited to patients who achieved a blood level of 10–29 ng/ml, the combined residual group of 14 patients showed a 93% significant response rate. In the author's current bupropion study, 300 mg/day of slow-release bupropion is being given in an open design for an 8-week period. Preliminary results indicate that patients with bipolar depression and atypical depression have a significantly better response than those with "typical depression," both in HDRS score reduction ($F = 5.57$, $P < .01$) and in BDI score reduction ($F = 3.32$, $P < .05$).

Similarly, Haykal and Akiskal (1990) presented evidence from six rapid-cycling bipolar II patients that bupropion produced significant improvement for both depression and overall cycling rate. A case of monthly, unipolar, psychotic depression that had persisted for 33 months was shown to respond to 300 mg/day of bupropion plus 4 mg/day of trifluoperazine; an immediate recovery and full remission was maintained for more than 16 months (Schenck et al. 1992). More recently, Sachs and colleagues (1994) presented a study of 10 patients who met DSM-III-R criteria for bipolar disorder and major depression that compared the response to 300 mg/day of desipramine and up to 450 mg/day of bupropion. All patients were maintained on sufficient lithium to produce a level of at least .6 mEq/L. Although there were only 5 patients per group, the initial response rate was equivalent at 40%; however, 60% of the desipramine patients switched into mania during the course of follow-up, compared with only 20% of the bupropion patients. This study presents evidence for the added safety of bupropion in bipolar patients. Bupropion may thus appear to be particularly useful in the treatment of atypical and bipolar depression. Table 3–2 summarizes the clinical predictors of response to SSRIs and bupropion.

> *Case 3: Bipolar depression.*   A 61-year-old man presented with a worsening two-year history of depression, despite being on fluoxetine for almost 4 months. Previously, he had not responded to a short treatment trial with sertraline. He had significant and worsening symptoms of dysphoria, pessimism, anhedonia, crying spells, irritability, ambivalence, lack of motivation, loss of libido, and insomnia. The key to treatment was the patient's episodic history of 5–6-month stretches when he experienced particularly increased productivity; this was associated with the pressure to "make more money." He made more business deals and drove his car more erratically during this time. His speech was also pressured, and he spoke at an increased rate. After a presumed diagnosis of previously missed bipolar II depression (major depression with past hypomania), the patient was prescribed 300 mg/day of bupropion in divided doses. His HDRS score dropped by more than 75%, and his BDI score dropped by more than 67% within 2 weeks of treatment. Furthermore, his anxiety and insomnia scores were dramatically better; all improvements were then maintained. Residual symptoms included only minimal dysphoria, a feeling of incapacity, mild irritability, and loss of libido. These symptoms dissipated over the next 2 weeks, and by the end of 1 month, the patient was virtually devoid of symptoms.

Table 3–2. Clinical predictors of response in depression

Medication class	Medication	Symptoms of depression	Types of depression
SSRI	Fluoxetine	± Retardation	+ Melancholia ± Atypical ± Bipolar
SSRI	Sertraline	−	± Melancholia
SSRI	Paroxetine	±	±
SSRI	Fluvoxamine	+ Anxiety, insomnia	
		− Retardation, diurnal change	
Aminoketone	Bupropion		+ Atypical, bipolar

Note. + = good response; ± = moderate response; − = poor response; SSRI = selective serotonin reuptake inhibitor.

Indicators for Combination of Depression with Other Disorders

Major depression may be frequently associated with other psychiatric disorders, including obsessive-compulsive disorder (OCD), impulse disorder, panic, and generalized anxiety disorder. The presence of these additional disorders may frequently give an indication of the appropriate choice of an antidepressant.

Obsessive-Compulsive Disorder

There are many biological and clinical similarities between major depression and OCD. Both conditions have been related to disturbances in serotonin. Improvement has been dependent, particularly with OCD, on using serotonin-based treatments. For example, in one case report, Pato and Zohar (1991) reported that a patient's disorder of combined depression and OCD revealed a response pattern in which, initially, the depression (but not the OCD) improved with amitriptyline, an antidepressant not specific to serotonin. When the patient was switched to the serotonergic TCA clomipramine, complete remission of both conditions was attained. Second, depressive symptoms may be sensitive to changes in serotonin when response is established. Discontinuation of clomipramine after 5–27 months of treatment was more likely to lead to relapse of depression than of OCD (Pato et al. 1988). Finally, the temporary elimination of tryptophan (the precursor of serotonin) from patients' diets led to relapse of depressive symptoms, but not of OCD symptoms, in patients on stabilized treatments for a mean of 16 weeks (Barr et al. 1994). In this section, the use of antidepressants in the treatment of symptoms of major depression with OCD is given priority.

Fluoxetine.   Numerous successful trials of fluoxetine in the treatment of OCD have shown a range of improvement of 30%–35% in the standard Yale-Brown Obsessive-Compulsive Scale (Y-BOCS) in typical 4–8-week periods (Liebowitz et al. 1989; Pigott et al. 1990). Some of the earliest data were reported by Turner and colleagues (1985). The basis for this treatment was the serotonergic hypothesis of OCD (Yaryura-Tobias et al. 1977). Ten patients who met DSM-III criteria for OCD were administered up to 80 mg/day of fluoxetine over a 12-week trial. It should be noted that the usual antidepressant dose of fluoxetine is 20 mg/day with a maximum of 80 mg/day. Many researchers have found that with fluoxetine, higher doses than are needed to treat depression are required to treat OCD (Pigott 1991). During the 12-week period, HDRS scores dropped by 10.4 ($P < .01$), but there was no significant change in the Maudsley OCD Inventory. In a second open-label study (Frenkel et al. 1990), up to 80 mg/day of fluoxetine was administered to 10 patients with DSM-III-R OCD for up to 32 weeks. In the first 4 weeks, the HDRS score dropped by a mean of 7.3 ($P < .002$), but there was no significant change in scores on either the OCD severity scale or the Hamilton Anxiety Rating Scale (HARS). By 8 weeks, the HARS scores had dropped by 3.4 ($P < .007$) and OCD severity scale scores by 1.0 ($P < .03$). By the end of 32 weeks, there was little further improvement. The third paper (Hollander et al. 1991) indicated that in a series of 10 patients who met DSM-III-R criteria for OCD (of whom eight had additional depression diagnoses, four of which were major depression), the administration of up to 80 mg/day of fluoxetine led to worsening or lack of improvement of depression. Sixty percent experienced an increase in symptoms when their fluoxetine dose was increased; 80% showed improvement when TCAs were administered with fluoxetine; however, only 2 of the 10 patients showed worsening of OCD. Thus, both depression and OCD show response to fluoxetine, but patients with combined disorders may not remit to fluoxetine treatment alone. The most recent fluoxetine studies (Dominguez et al. 1994; Tollefson et al. 1994b) showed that, in contrast to depression (where 20–40 mg/day produced the best responses), the best dose response for OCD symptoms was probably 60 mg/day.

Sertraline. There have been three reports regarding the use of sertraline in OCD. The first of these studies used patients without symptoms of major depression and without significant HDRS scores (Jenike et al. 1990a). At 200 mg/day of sertraline for 10 weeks, there was no significant change in the Y-BOCS (–9.6%). It is possible that because there may be a "window" in clinical response to sertraline, this dose may have been too high to produce a clinical response. The 200 mg/day dose is the maximum allowed by the FDA, and the related possible minimum and maximum plasma levels for response have been described (Goodnick 1994). The second study (Chouinard et al. 1990) reported the results of 180 mg/day of sertraline for 8 weeks of treatment. The drop in Y-BOCS was 16.2% (this was significantly greater than placebo, $P = .05$). The third study looked at 50–200 mg/day of sertraline for 12 weeks (Greist et al. 1995). Nondepressed patients with OCD responded well after only 2 weeks of therapy. Pooled results indicated a mean decrease in the Y-BOCS of 5.57 (23.4%) in the sertraline patients and of 3.41 (14.6%) in the placebo group. Thus, sertraline may be useful in patients with both depression and OCD, but conclusive evidence is lacking. The most recent report on OCD showed that higher doses than those typically used for depression (e.g., 200 mg/day) produced the best response (Dominguez et al. 1994); however, this level of response appears much less frequently than with fluoxetine, a less serotonin-specific reuptake inhibitor.

Case 4: Major depression with OCD.   A 29-year-old woman had a history of atypical depression associated with hyperphagia and hypersomnia and had responded to 300 mg/day of bupropion. After maintaining improvement for 2 years, the medication was stopped. In the winter of 1993, however, the patient experienced a relapse of major depression; this time, it was associated with obsessive thoughts of harming her fiancé. She became phobic from the "fear" of finding a knife when emptying a dishwasher, and consequently stopped doing such chores. There were also associated fears of getting too close to people. She had developed a habit of repeatedly pulling on her eyelashes. Such thoughts and behaviors were upsetting her professional and personal life. Bupropion treatment was again started, but it did not have any impact on her depression or other symptoms this time. She was then given 50 mg/day of sertraline; its serotonergic specificity had the potential to alleviate the proposed 5-HT basis for OCD. Three weeks after beginning treatment, the severity (i.e., intensity and frequency) of her obsessive thoughts decreased by 50%. Her eyelash-pulling habit substantially diminished, and her paralysis had decreased enough to let her exercise again. Her fear of finding knives was also resolved, allowing her to put her residence back in order. Approximately 2 months after beginning treatment, her obsessive thoughts had almost disappeared completely, and the major depression had subsided. She was able to successfully make and carry out her wedding plans.

Paroxetine.   Literature on the treatment of OCD with the highly specific SSRI, paroxetine, is minimal. Dominguez and colleagues (1994) found that 34% of patients appeared to respond after 6 months of open-label treatment, somewhat lower than that for fluoxetine (40%–48%). Furthermore, there may be a dose-response relationship similar to the other SSRIs, in which higher doses are needed to treat OCD (40–60 mg/day) than depression (20 mg/day). Further, Wheadon and colleagues (1993) recently reported that in a 12-week double-blind protocol, 40 or 60 mg/day of paroxetine, but not 20 mg/day, produced significant improvement over placebo in the treatment of OCD. Improvement in the Y-BOCS was similar in 20 mg and placebo groups (both 13.7%); for 40 mg/day, it was 21.6%. Only a dosage greater than indicated for depression (20–50 mg/day) of 60 mg/day showed a response rate of 31.3%

Fluvoxamine.   There is presently a wide body of literature regarding the use of fluvoxamine in OCD. In this section, the focus is on selected papers. Perse and colleagues (1987) studied 20 patients with DSM-III-R OCD with a mean HDRS score of approximately 14. After 8 weeks of a maximum of 150 mg of fluvoxamine twice a day, there were significant reductions in the Maudsley OCD Inventory (2.36, –14.6%, $P < .02$), the HARS scores (4.40, –36.4%, $P < .002$), and the HDRS scores (4.51, –32.3%, $P < .007$). Goodman and colleagues have published two studies on the use of fluvoxamine in OCD. The first (Goodman et al. 1989) reported results on 42 patients who met DSM-III criteria for OCD; patients with depressive symptoms were included if they were considered to be following the onset of OCD, and if their depression was judged to be "secondary" to OCD. Accepted patients were separated into "depressed" (HDRS score ≥ 20) and "nondepressed" (HDRS score < 20) categories. In this double-blind comparison with placebo, 10 patients in each treatment group were determined to have concurrent major depression. By the end of the 6–8-week period, patients were receiving a mean of 255 mg/day of fluvoxamine or 274 mg/day of placebo. Patients receiving fluvoxamine experienced a reduction from 27 to 19 in their Y-BOCS (–30%, $P < .05$). Forty-two percent of patients were found to be significantly improved on fluvoxamine. HDRS scores were significantly reduced during the therapy period; however, after treatment, there was no significant difference between drug and placebo in rate of significant improvement. The response of OCD patients was not related to baseline HDRS scores in either group; also, the average reduction in HDRS score was not different between OCD patients who did and did not respond. In a further study of Goodman and colleagues (1990), fluvoxamine was found to be significantly better than the noradrenergic TCA desipramine in reducing both OCD and secondary depression severity. Overall, the decline in the Y-BOCS was −29% for fluvoxamine and 0% for desipramine, with a corresponding rate of significant response of 11 of 21 (52%) for fluvoxamine and two of 19 (11%) for desipramine. A further analysis, however, showed that fluvoxamine, not desipramine, was effective in the treatment of depressive symptoms in patients with OCD. In this comparison of up to 300 mg/day of each medication, after 8 weeks the HDRS scores decreased by 12% in desipramine patients and by 65% in fluvoxamine patients. Additionally, patients with OCD and severe depression responded less favorably in terms of OCD than those who did not have associated depression. Patients who experienced an improvement in OCD symptoms had lower baseline mean HDRS scores (20.9 versus 31.3, respectively). Correspondingly, there were more OCD patients who responded to fluvoxamine in the nondepressed group than in the depressed group (71% versus 43%, respectively). Jenike and colleagues (1990b) replicated these findings on the administration of a maximum of 300 mg/day of fluvoxamine for a period of 10 weeks. The Y-BOCS fell by 3.8 (−15%, $P < .001$), and the National Institute of Mental Health Global OCD fell by 1.9 (−22%, $P < .001$). There was no relationship between improvement on the Y-BOCS and the baseline HDRS score ($r = .21$, $P = NS$). It was further stated that the effect size in amelioration of OCD was reversed from that of 5-HT selectivity. The effect size was greatest for clomipramine (1.53), followed by fluoxetine (1.34), fluvoxamine (1.09), and sertraline (.80). Therefore, the presence of OCD together with depressive symptoms should lead the clinician to consider the SSRIs, and, in particular, those SSRIs (fluvoxamine and fluoxetine) that are less 5-HT specific in order to maximize response of both disorders.

Anxiety and Other Clinical Characteristics

The SSRIs have been used in the treatment of both anger attacks and panic disorder. Fava and colleagues (1991, 1993) demonstrated that "anger attacks" (as "sudden spells of anger resembling panic attacks but lacking the affects of fear and anxiety") respond to fluoxetine (p. 275). As part of their initial study, six of nine patients with both DSM-III-R major depression and anger attacks were cleared of these attacks after treatment with fluoxetine for at least 8 weeks. In the follow-up study, 71% of another group of patients with DSM-III-R major depressive disorder indicated disappearance of these attacks after 8 weeks of open treatment with 20 mg/day of fluoxetine. In a comparison with those with major depression but without anger attacks, there was a trend for greater overall improvement in the group with anger attacks.

> *Case 5: Anger attacks.* A 26-year-old woman had been experiencing "anger attacks" at the time of interview. These attacks (which came in bursts of up to 5 per day, every 2 weeks) came on suddenly and provoked behavior "like that of a 5-year-old." The state, according to her, was so intense that when it ended, "it was like waking up from a dream." She described the loss of control as an "impulse" to hurt her boyfriend. These brief attacks were associated with dysphoria, crying spells, self-hate, anorexia, decreased concentration, anhedonia, and decreased thought. The patient experienced neither obsession nor compulsion. Fluoxetine, at a dose of 20 mg/day, produced significant resolution of these anger attacks. Within 2 weeks, the frequency was only 1 per week, and the patient also experienced simultaneous improvement of her major depression symptoms. The attacks disappeared within 1 month.

Panic and Posttraumatic Stress Disorder

In patients with panic disorder, there have been positive published results for fluoxetine, particularly at low doses (Gorman et al. 1987; Schneier et al. 1990). Many patients with panic disorders cannot tolerate even 20 mg/day (Louie et al. 1993). At a dose of 20–80 mg/day, fluoxetine has been found effective in the treatment of posttraumatic stress disorder (Nagy et al. 1993). Finally, fluvoxamine at 100–150 mg/day has been reported to be effective in the treatment of panic disorder (Den Boer et al. 1987, 1988). Thus, although not a predictor of response, patients with major depressive disorder and simultaneous panic attacks may respond well to an SSRI. Most recently, there have been several reports concerning panic disorder and SSRIs: sertraline (1994), paroxetine (1995), and fluvoxamine (1995—three reports). Gorman and Wolkow reported that sertraline at a dose of 50–200 mg/day given double-blind versus placebo to 320 patients for 12 weeks in pooled data reduced panic attacks by 90% (placebo rate of reduction = 50%). Limited symptom attacks were reduced by 67% (versus placebo rate of 20%). The results were not dose-dependent (i.e., reductions in panic attacks were as significant for 50 mg as for 200 mg). The report on paroxetine in 278 patients indicated that statistical differences for up to 40 mg/day in severity and frequency of panic attacks were significantly better than placebo (Steiner et al. 1995). de Beurs and colleagues (1995) recently published results on use of fluvoxamine on a double-blind basis in 96 patients of up to 150 mg/day versus placebo for treatment of panic disorder with agoraphobia for 12 weeks. The addition of fluvoxamine with exposure produced superior efficacy over placebo plus exposure ($P < .001$) or exposure alone ($P = .003$). At the 1995 American Psychiatric Association Annual Meeting, fluvoxamine in conjunction with cognitive behavior was shown in a 12-week protocol to earliest treatment effect and largest response at week 12 of 83% in 190 patients in contrast to placebo or either treatment alone (Simpson et al. 1995). Finally, in contrast to placebo in a double-blind program, 26 patients treated with fluvoxamine showed a significant decrease in rate of CCK-4-induced panic attacks from 76% to 29% (van Megen et al. 1995).

Table 3–3 summarizes the prediction of response to SSRIs in depression accompanied by other anxiety disorders.

Table 3–3.   Treatment of depression with other associated problems

SSRI	OCD	Panic	Other
Fluoxetine	+ +	+ (low dose)	+ (PTSD)
Sertraline	+	+	
Paroxetine	+	+	
Fluvoxamine	+ +	+	

Note.   SSRI = selective serotonin reuptake inhibitor; OCD = obsessive-compulsive disorder; PTSD = posttraumatic stress disorder.

Summary: Guidelines on Predictors to New Antidepressants

In this section, some possible indicators have been seen that require further replication to be established for routine clinical application. For biochemical predictors, it appears that evidence for serotonin deficiency, whether of platelet or neuroendocrine origin, may lead one to successfully treat a patient with the most potent SSRIs (i.e., sertraline and paroxetine). A positive DST result may also be associated with a better response to sertraline or trazodone. With regard to clinical predictors, patients with psychomotor retardation may be more successfully treated with fluoxetine, whereas those with agitation may have better results with fluvoxamine. Melancholic patients respond well to fluoxetine, whereas atypical and bipolar depressed patients may benefit most from bupropion. In terms of depression with other associated disorders, patients with OCD and major depression may benefit most from fluvoxamine and fluoxetine, the relatively less specific SSRIs. Fluoxetine may be best in treating "anger attacks," panic attacks, and posttraumatic stress syndrome. Because of the difficulty with fluoxetine's side effects, fluvoxamine may be better in the overall response of panic attacks to SSRIs.

References

American Psychiatric Association Task Force on Laboratory Tests in Psychiatry: The dexamethasone suppression test: an overview of its current status in psychiatry. Am J Psychiatry 144:1253–1262, 1987

Baldassano CF, Sachs GS, Stoll AL, et al: Paroxetine for bipolar depression (NR101), in New Research Program and Abstracts: American Psychiatric Association 148th Annual Meeting, Miami, Florida, May 20–25, 1995. Washington, DC, American Psychiatric Association, 1995, pp 81–82

Barr LC, Goodman WK, McDougle CJ, et al: Tryptophan depletion in patients with obsessive-compulsive disorder who respond to serotonin reuptake inhibitors. Arch Gen Psychiatry 51:309–317, 1994

Beasley CM, Sayler ME, Bosomworth JC, et al: High-dose fluoxetine: efficacy and activating-sedating effects in agitated and retarded depression. J Clin Psychopharmacol 11:166–174, 1991

Bowden CL, Schatzberg AF, Rosenbaum A, et al: Fluoxetine and desipramine in major depressive disorder. J Clin Psychopharmacol 13:305–311, 1993

Cain JW: Poor response to fluoxetine: underlying depression, serotonergic overstimulation, or a "therapeutic window." J Clin Psychiatry 53:272–277, 1992

Carroll BJ, Feinberg M, Greden JF, et al: A specific laboratory test for the diagnosis of melancholia: standardization, validation, and clinical utility. Arch Gen Psychiatry 38:15–22, 1981

Celada P, Dolera M, Alvarez E, et al: Effects of acute and chronic treatment with fluvoxamine on extracellular and platelet serotonin in the blood of major depressive patients. Relationship to clinical outcome. J Affect Disord 25:243–250, 1992

Chouinard G, Goodman W, Greist J, et al: Results of a double-blind placebo-controlled trial of a new serotonin uptake inhibitor, sertraline, in the treatment of obsessive compulsive disorder. Psychopharmacol Bull 26:279–284, 1990

Cohn JB, Collins G, Ashbrook E, et al: A comparison of fluoxetine, imipramine and placebo in patients with bipolar depressive disorder. Int Clin Psychopharmacol 4:313–322, 1989

Danish University Antidepressant Group: Paroxetine: a selective serotonin reuptake inhibitor showing better tolerance, but weaker antidepressant effect than clomipramine in a controlled multicenter study. J Affect Disord 18:289–299, 1990

De Bellis MD, Geracioti TD Jr, Altemus M, et al: Cerebrospinal fluid monoamine metabolites in fluoxetine-treated patients with major depression and in healthy volunteers. Biol Psychiatry 33:636–641, 1993

de Beurs E, van Balkom AJLM, Lange A, et al: Treatment of panic disorder with agoraphobia: comparison of fluvoxamine, placebo, and psychological panic management combined with exposure and of exposure in vivo alone. Am J Psychiatry 152:683–691, 1995

Delgado PL, Price LH, Charney DS, et al: Efficacy of fluvoxamine in treatment-refractory depression. J Affect Disord 15:55–60, 1988

Den Boer JA, Westenberg HGM, Kamerbeek WDJ, et al: Effect of serotonin uptake inhibitors in anxiety disorders: a double-blind comparison of clomipramine and fluvoxamine. Int Clin Psychopharmacol 2:21–32, 1987

Den Boer JA, Westenberg HGM: Effect of a serotonin and noradrenaline uptake inhibitor in panic disorder: a double-blind comparative study with fluvoxamine and maprotiline. Int Clin Psychopharmacol 3:59–74, 1988

Dominguez RA, Gandara JDL, Knowles L: Dissociation between pharma-codynamics and efficacy in obsessive-compulsive disorder (OCD). Paper presented at annual meeting of the American College of Clinical Pharmacology, Washington, DC, April 1994

Falk J, Trestman RL, Mitropoulou V, et al: Serotonin and prediction of fluoxetine response time (NR75), in New Research Program and Abstracts: American Psychiatric Association 148th Annual Meeting, Miami, Florida, May 20–25, 1995. Washington, DC, APA, 1995, p 74

Fava M, Rosenbaum JF, McCarthy M, et al: Anger attacks in depressed outpatients and their response to fluoxetine. Psychopharmacol Bull 27:275–279, 1991

Fava M, Rosenbaum JF, Pava JA, et al: Anger attacks in unipolar depression, I: clinical correlates and response to fluoxetine treatment. Am J Psychiatry 150:1158–1168, 1993

Ferris RM, Cooper BR, Maxwell RA: Studies of bupropion's mechanism of antidepressant activity. J Clin Psychiatry 44:5 (sec 2), 74–78, 1983

Gasperini M, Gatti F, Bellini L, et al: Perspectives in clinical psychopharmacology of amitriptyline and fluvoxamine. Pharmacopsychiatry 26:186–192, 1992

Golden RN, Rudorfer MV, Sherer MA, et al: Bupropion in depression, I: biochemical effects and clinical response. Arch Gen Psychiatry 45:139–143, 1988

Goodman WK, Price LH, Rasmussen SA, et al: Efficacy of fluvoxamine in obsessive-compulsive disorder. Arch Gen Psychiatry 46:36–44, 1989

Goodman WK, Price LH, Delgado PL, et al: Specificity of serotonin reuptake inhibitors in the treatment of obsessive-compulsive disorder. Arch Gen Psychiatry 47:577–585, 1990

Goodnick PJ: Blood levels and acute response to bupropion. Am J Psychiatry 149:399–400, 1992

Goodnick PJ: Pharmacokinetics optimization of therapy with newer antidepressants. Clin Pharmacokinet 27:307–330, 1994

Goodnick PJ, Extein IL: Bupropion and fluoxetine in depressive subtypes. Ann Clin Psychiatry 1:119–122, 1989

Goodnick PJ, Henry J, Kumar A: Neurochemistry and paroxetine response in major depression. Biol Psychiatry 37:417–419, 1995

Goodnick PJ, Sandoval R, Brickman A, et al: Bupropion treatment of fluoxetine-resistant chronic fatigue syndrome. Biol Psychiatry 32:834–838, 1992

Gorman JM, Leibowitz MR, Fyer AJ, et al: An open trial of fluoxetine in the treatment of panic attacks. J Clin Psychopharmacol 7:329–332, 1987

Gorman J, Wolkow R: Sertraline as a treatment for panic disorder. CINP, Washington, DC, 1994

Greist J, Chouinard G, DuBoff E, et al: Double-blind parallel comparison of three doses of sertraline and placebo in outpatients with obsessive-compulsive disorder. Arch Gen Psychiatry 52;289–295, 1995

Haykal RF, Akiskal HS: Bupropion as a promising approach to rapid cycling bipolar II patients. J Clin Psychiatry 51:450–455, 1990

Hollander E, Mullen L, DeCaria CM, et al: Obsessive-compulsive disorder, depression, and fluoxetine. J Clin Psychiatry 52:418–422, 1991

Hollander E, Stein DJ, DeCaria CM, et al: A pilot study of biological predictors of treatment outcome in obsessive-compulsive disorder. Biol Psychiatry 33:747–749, 1993

Jenike MA, Baer L, Summergrad P, et al: Sertraline in obsessive-compulsive disorder: a double-blind comparison with placebo. Am J Psychiatry 147:923–928, 1990a

Jenike MA, Hyman S, Baer L, et al: A controlled trial of fluvoxamine in obsessive-compulsive disorder. Am J Psychiatry 147:1209–1215, 1990b

Johnson MR, Lydiard RB, Morton WA, et al: Effect of fluvoxamine, imipramine and placebo on catecholamine function in depressed outpatients. J Psychiatry Res 27:161–172, 1993

Kasper S, Voll G, Vieira A, et al: Response to total sleep deprivation before and during treatment with fluvoxamine or maprotiline in patients with major depression: results of a double-blind study. Pharmacopsychiatry 23:135–142, 1990

Kasper S, Fugar J, Moller H-J: Comparative efficacy of antidepressants. Drugs 43(suppl 2):11–23, 1992

Kremer HPH, Goekoop JG, Van Kempen GMJ: Clinical use of the determination of serotonin in whole blood. J Clin Psychopharmacol 10:83–87, 1990

Laakmann G, Blaschke D, Engel R, et al: Fluoxetine versus amitriptyline in the treatment of depressed out-patients. Br J Psychiatry 153(suppl 3):64–68, 1988

Liebowitz MR, Hollander E, Schneier F, et al: Fluoxetine treatment of obsessive-compulsive disorder: an open clinical trial. J Clin Psychopharmacol 9:423–427, 1989

Louie AK, Lewis TB, Lannon RA: Use of low-dose fluoxetine in major depression and panic disorder. J Clin Psychiatry 54:435–438, 1993

Lu R-B, Ko H-C, Huang C-C, et al: The relationship of monoamine systems to fluoxetine responsiveness in depressed patients (abstract no 84). Biol Psychiatry 31:98A, 1992

Malone KM, Thase ME, Dealy RS, et al: Biological treatment effects on serotonin responsivity and outcome in major depression. Biol Psychiatry 33:80A, #161, 1993

Moller SE, Bech P, Bjerrum H, et al: Plasma ratio tryptophan/neutral amino acids in relation to clinical response to paroxetine and clomipramine in patients with major depression. J Affect Disord 18:59–66, 1990

Moscovitch A, Wiseman RL, Goldberg MS, et al: A double-blind, placebo-controlled study of sertraline in the treatment of outpatients with SAD (NR440), in New Research Program and Abstracts: American Psychiatric Association 148th Annual Meeting, Miami, Florida, May 20–25, 1995. Washington, DC, American Psychiatric Association, 1995, pp 173–174

Muck-Seler D, Jakovljevic M, Deanovic Z: Effect of antidepressant treatment on platelet 5-HT content and relations to therapeutic outcome in unipolar depressive patients. J Affect Disord 23:157–164, 1991

Murdoch D, McTavish D: Sertraline: a review of its pharmacodynamic and pharmacokinetic properties, therapeutic potential in depressive illness, and prospective role in treatment of obsessive-compulsive disorder. Drugs 44:604–624, 1992

Nagy LM, Morgan CA III, Southwick SM, et al: Open prospective trial of fluoxetine for posttraumatic stress disorder. J Clin Psychopharmacol 13: 107–113, 1993

Nathan RS, Perel JM, Pollock BG, et al: The role of neuropharmacologic selectively in antidepressant action: fluvoxamine versus desipramine. J Clin Psychiatry 51:367–372, 1990

Palmer KJ, Benfield P: Fluvoxamine: an overview of its pharmacological properties and review of its therapeutic potential in nondepressive disorders. CNS Drugs 1:57–87, 1994

Pande AC, Sayler ME: Severity of depression and response to fluoxetine. Int Clin Psychopharmacol 8:243–245, 1993

Pato MT, Zohar J: Clomipramine in the treatment of obsessive-compulsive disorder, in Current Treatments of Obsessive-Compulsive Disorder. Edited by Pato MT, Zohar J. Washington, DC, and London, American Psychiatric Press, 1991, pp. 13–28

Pato MT, Zohar-Kadouch R, Zohar J, et al: Return of symptoms after discontinuation of clomipramine in patients with obsessive-compulsive disorder. Am J Psychiatry 145:12, 1521–1525, 1988

Perse TL, Greist JH, Jefferson JW, et al: Fluvoxamine treatment of obsessive-compulsive disorder. Am J Psychiatry 144:1543–1548, 1987

Peselow ED, Lautin A, Wolkin A, et al: The dexamethasone suppression test and response to placebo. J Clin Psychopharmacol 6:286–291, 1986

Peselow ED, Stanley M, Filippi A-M, et al: The predictive value of the dexamethasone suppression test. Br J Psychiatry 155:667–672, 1989

Pigott TA: Fluoxetine in the treatment of obsessive-compulsive disorder, in Current Treatments of Obsessive-Compulsive Disorder. Edited by Pato MT, Zohar J. Washington, DC, and London, American Psychiatric Press, 1991, pp 29–44

Pigott TA, Pato MT, Bernstein SE, et al: Controlled comparisons of clomipramine and fluoxetine in the treatment of obsessive-compulsive disorder. Arch Gen Psychiatry 47:926–932, 1990

Price LH, Charney DS, Delgado PL, et al: Effects of desipramine and fluvoxamine treatment on the prolactin response to tryptophan. Arch Gen Psychiatry 46:625–631, 1989

Quitkin FM, Stewart JW, McGrath P, et al: Phenelzine versus imipramine in probable atypical depression: defining syndrome boundaries of selective MAO responders. Am J Psychiatry 145:306–312, 1988

Reimherr FW, Wood DR, Byerley B, et al: Characteristics of responders to fluoxetine. Psycopharmacol Bull 20:70–72, 1984

Reimherr FW, Chouinard G, Cohn CK, et al: Antidepressant efficacy of sertraline: a double-blind, placebo- and amitriptyline-controlled, multicenter comparison study in outpatients with major depression. J Clin Psychiatry 51[12(suppl B)]:18–27, 1990

Renshaw PF, Guimaraes AR, Fava M, et al: Accumulation of fluoxetine and norfluoxetine in human brain during therapeutic administration. Am J Psychiatry 149:1592–1594, 1992

Ribeiro SCM, Tandon R, Grunhaus L, et al: The DST as a predictor of outcome in depression: a meta-analysis. Am J Psychiatry 150:1618–1629, 1993

Rosenbaum JF, Fava M, Pava JA, et al: Anger attacks in unipolar depression; part 2: neuroendocrine correlates and changes following treatment. Am J Psychiatry 150:1164–1168, 1993

Rosenthal J, Hemlock C, Hellerstein DJ, et al: A preliminary study of serotonergic antidepressants in treatment of dysthymia. Prog Neuropsychopharmacol Biol Psychiatry 16:933–941, 1992

Sachs GS, Stoll AL, Lafer B, et al: Bupropion versus desipramine in bipolar depression: a double-blind comparison of acute and maintenance effects. J Clin Psychiatry 55:391–393, 1994

Salzman C, Jimerson D, Vasile R, et al: Response to SSRI antidepressants correlates with reduction in plasma HVA: pilot study. Biol Psychiatry 34:569–571, 1993

Schildkraut JJ, Schatzberg AF, Samson JA, et al: Norepinephrine output and metabolism in depressed patients during anti-depressant treatment. Clin Neuropharmacol 15(suppl 1A):323A–324A, 1992

Schneier FR, Liebowitz MR, Davies SO, et al: Fluoxetine in panic disorder. J Clin Psychopharmacol 10:119–121, 1990

Simon JS, Evans DL, Nemeroff CB: The dexamethasone suppression test and antidepressant response in major depression. J Psychiatr Res 21:313–317, 1987

Simpson RJ, Sharp DM, Power KG: Cost effectiveness of fluvoxamine, placebo, and cognitive behavior therapy alone and in combination in the treatment of panic disorder (NR357), in New Research Program and Abstracts: American Psychiatric Association 148th Annual Meeting, Miami, Florida, May 20–25, 1995. Washington, DC, American Psychiatric Association, 1995, p 151

Simpson SG, DePaulo JR: Fluoxetine treatment of bipolar II depression. J Clin Psychopharmacol 11:52–54, 1991

Spitzer RL, Endicott J, Robins E: Research Diagnostic Criteria: rationale and reliability. Arch Gen Psychiatry 35:773–782, 1978

Steiner M, Oakes R, Gergel IP: A fixed dose study of paroxetine and placebo in the treatment of panic disorder (NR355), in New Research Program and Abstracts: American Psychiatric Association, 148th Annual Meeting, Miami, Florida, May 20–25, 1995. Washington, DC, American Psychiatric Association, 1995, p 150

Stratta P, Bolino F, Cupillari M, et al: A double-blind parallel study comparing fluoxetine with imipramine in the treatment of atypical depression. Int Clin Psychopharmacol 6:193–196, 1991

Taneri Z, Kohler R: Fluoxetine versus nomifensine in outpatients with neurotic or reactive depressive disorder. Int Clin Psychopharmacol 4 (supp 1):57–61, 1989

Tollefson GD: Do [^{3}H]-imipramine platelet studies reflect treatment outcomes of major depression-agitated subtype? Presented New Research, Annual Meeting, American Psychiatric Association, Philadelphia, PA, May 1994

Tollefson GD, Holman SL: Analysis of the Hamilton depression rating scale factors from a double-blind, placebo-controlled trial of fluoxetine in geriatric major depression. Int Clin Psychopharmacol 8:253–259, 1993

Tollefson GD, Holman SL, Sayler ME, et al: Fluoxetine, placebo, and tricyclic antidepressants in major depression with and without anxious features. J Clin Psychiatry 55:50–59, 1994a

Tollefson GD, Rampey Jr AH, Potvin JH, et al: A multicenter investigation of fixed-dose fluoxetine in the treatment of obsessive-compulsive disorder. Arch Gen Psychiatry 51:559–567, 1994b

van Megen HJGM, Westenberg HGM, den Boer JA: Effect of the selective serotonin reuptake inhibitor fluvoxamine on CCK-4 induced panic attacks. Biol Psychiatry 37:619, 1995

Wheadon DE, Bushnell WD, Steiner M: A fixed dose comparison of 20, 40, or 60 mg paroxetine to placebo in the treatment of obsessive-compulsive disorder. Presented at Annual Meeting, American College of Neuropsychopharmacology, Honolulu, Hawaii, December 1993

Yaryura-Tobias JA, Bebrian RJ, Neziroglu FA, et al: Obsessive-compulsive disorders as a serotonergic deficit. Res Commun Psychol Psychiatry Behav 2:279–286, 1977

CHAPTER 4

Lithium

James W. Jefferson, M.D.

"If you undulate, we medicate."

—*University of Wisconsin Lithium Clinic, 1974*

*T*he therapeutic promise of lithium reached such epic proportion in the 1970s that our motto was only partially in jest. Yet even then, it was well recognized that bipolar patients sometimes resisted the elemental charm of lithium. A rudimentary rule of response prediction was also evident early on, namely, that the more "classic" or "pure" the presentation, the greater the likelihood of a favorable response to lithium. Since then, the quest for a highly reliable response predictor has continued. In 1980, the prediction of lithium response was the subject of an international symposium, the proceedings of which were published in 1983 (DuFour et al. 1983). A search in December 1993 of the Lithium Information Center database revealed 535 references with the subject heading "response prediction."

Unfortunately, however, there are a number of important response prediction issues that have not been resolved. Some are general and others apply more specifically to lithium. For example, does dysphoric or mixed mania predict a poor response to lithium but not to alternatives such as carbamazepine and valproate, or does it predict a nonspecific reduced responsiveness to all therapeutic interventions? Comorbid substance abuse or personality disorder has been associated with poorer treatment outcome, but there appears to be nothing unique to lithium in this regard. Whereas one could easily predict a less than ideal response to lithium in a bipolar, alcoholic patient with borderline personality disorder, the same would also be true for other mood stabilizers.

Other generic issues include the definition of response and nonresponse and inconsistencies in such definitions across studies. For example, in depression studies, a response is often defined as a 50% or greater reduction in Hamilton Depression Rating Scale score. Obviously, this definition includes patients who respond both partially and fully. With regard to lithium prophylaxis, response could be defined in terms of no further episodes, fewer episodes, shortened episode duration, reduced episode severity, and combinations thereof. Comparing outcomes of response prediction studies is somewhat clouded by these definitional vagaries.

Another unresolved issue is whether patients who do not respond to lithium but respond to an alternate treatment share characteristics that would have predictive value in choosing treatment for patients not previously exposed to any mood stabilizer. The inclusion of patients previously treated (successfully or unsuccessfully) with lithium but never exposed to the new drug has often been a design bias in studies comparing a newer drug to lithium.

Another major confounder in the response prediction field is noncompliance. Is an outcome predictor successful because it predicts which patients will take the medication or because the medication, once taken, will be effective? For example, alcohol abuse is associated with poor compliance, but would a compliant bipolar alcoholic patient respond well to lithium? Or are there features inherent to this comorbidity that interfere with treatment response even in the presence of consistently adequate serum lithium levels? Aagaard and Vestergaard (1990) reported that noncompliance with prophylactic lithium therapy was predicted by a history of substance abuse and prior hospitalizations, whereas nonresponse in lithium-adherent patients was predicted by being young, female, and having a chronic clinical course. Difficulty in separating noncompliance from pharmacologic nonresponse continues to muddy the interpretation of outcome data.

Other unresolved issues include whether mood state influences the reliability of an outcome predictor. For example, could test A predict a favorable antimanic response to drug B if administered while the patient is euthymic but fail to do so if administered during a manic episode? Can one assume that failure to respond to lithium during the first manic episode accurately predicts failure to respond during all subsequent episodes? More broadly, is response or nonresponse a constant across episodes, or might there be inconsistencies that would wreak havoc with response prediction studies (Carroll 1979)? For example, Stokes and colleagues (1971) found that response to lithium sometimes varied across episodes of mania in the same patient. Reasons for such variability could include inconsistent compliance, the course of the episode in which treatment was initiated, the severity of the episode, the use of concomitant medications, and the environment in which the episode was treated.

Shapiro and colleagues (1989) point out analysis flaws in many of the studies of long-term maintenance of bipolar disorder. They stress the need to consider factors such as wellness duration (rather than treatment failure alone) and to properly evaluate patients who withdraw from studies for reasons other than episode recurrence. For example, the original report of the National Institute of Mental Health Collaborative Study comparing lithium, imipramine, and a combination of the two for prevention of recurrences in bipolar and unipolar affective disorder found no significant differences among treatments in bipolar patients if the index episode was depression (Prien et al. 1984). When Shapiro and colleagues (1989) reanalyzed these data using survival analysis statistics, however, they found that the combination of lithium and imipramine was more effective than either drug alone.

Reasons for the apparent reduction in lithium's effectiveness in recent years must be addressed. Grof and colleagues (1993) suggest that lithium never "stopped working" and that the apparent erosion in benefit (from 70%–80% in the 1960s and 1970s to 20%–30% in the 1980s and 1990s) is mostly an artifact of patient selection. Elsewhere, Grof and colleagues (1983b) succinctly state that "the advent of lithium has significantly increased the number of people diagnosed as manic depressives" (p. 52). Included in this group are both correctly and incorrectly diagnosed patients. They further state that "as with any other approach, the percentage of success one achieves with lithium treatment is a function of how carefully one selects the patients likely to benefit. Most of the patients placed on lithium today do not suffer from the condition for which lithium was originally proven effective" (Grof et al. 1993, p. 18).

To further complicate matters, one must also consider problems inherent in response prediction when treatment is less than 100% effective. If the optimal response rate in a carefully defined, highly compliant population is 90%, then searching that population for response predictors is likely to be more rewarding than doing the same in a population in which the best possible outcome is 30%. As discussed later in this chapter, Grof and colleagues were able to correctly predict outcome in 83% of patients in a prospective maintenance study using six variables in a carefully defined population (Grof et al. 1983a).

In this chapter we critically evaluate what is known about predicting response to lithium. Emphasis is placed on response prediction in acute mania, acute depression, and long-term maintenance, and the exclusion of less well-studied conditions outside the area of mood disorders.

Acute Mania

Demographic and Clinical Predictors

The literature is fraught with inconsistencies when it comes to predicting an acute antimanic response to lithium. Miller and colleagues (1991), in a retrospective review of 53 bipolar manic patients (which included 13 patients who did not respond), found that response could not be predicted by the presence of features such as paranoia, elation, grandiosity, delusions, hallucinations, irritability, agitation, and aggressiveness. Patients who responded as well as patients who did not respond both had mean serum lithium levels slightly above 0.9 mEq/L.

Similar results were obtained by Taylor and Abrams (1981) who evaluated 111 manic patients (56% of whom responded and 44% of whom did not) treated with a variety of approaches but predominantly with lithium and neuroleptics. After examining a broad range of demographic and clinical features, they found "no adequate predictors of short-term treatment response in mania" (p. 800). For example, the response in euphoric, grandiose manics did not differ from those who were paranoid-destructive. Swann and colleagues (1986) also found that irritable-paranoid manics did not respond less well to lithium.

These studies are in contrast to research by Murphy and Biegel (1974), who found a poorer treatment response in their paranoid-destructive manic patients. These patients also had more depressive symptoms accompanying the mania, so perhaps the dysphoria, rather than the paranoia, predicted poor response.

Cohen and colleagues (1989), in addition to nicely summarizing the conflicting literature, looked for response predictors in 44 consecutively admitted manic patients. Patients who did and did not respond to lithium did not have significantly different scores on either the Brief Psychiatric Rating Scale (BPRS) or the Manic Rating Scale (MRS) upon admission with regard to total score as well as most subscale scores. The exception was that patients who did not respond had a higher degree of depressive symptomatology. The only other significant difference was an earlier age at onset in the patients who did not respond as opposed to patients who did (19.3 versus 30.3 years, respectively). As the authors readily acknowledged, the presence of only four patients in the nonresponse group limited conclusions that could be drawn from the study.

Episode Severity

Severe manic episodes are alleged to be less responsive to lithium, although this may be due in part to an artifact of limited treatment duration. Severely ill patients may not be able to comply with treatment long enough to allow lithium to become effective. On the other hand, Swann and colleagues (1986) treated 18 manic patients with lithium in the absence of antipsychotic drugs and found a poorer outcome in patients with more severe mania, anxiety, and depression ratings (although psychotic symptoms did not predict poor outcome). Practically speaking, severe manic episodes will require the use of ancillary treatments such as antipsychotics or benzodiazepines, and whether responsiveness to lithium is really different is of little interest to clinicians. It is generally agreed that once an episode has stabilized, efforts should be made to taper and stop medications other than lithium, regardless of initial episode severity.

Rapid cycling.   Rapid cycling has been arbitrarily defined as four or more episodes of mania or depression per year. Although some patients cycle rapidly from the onset of illness, far more become rapid cyclers as the illness progresses. Studies have found that up to 20% of bipolar patients experience rapid cycling and that the condition is more common in women. Although rapid cyclers generally respond poorly to lithium, focus has usually been on prophylactic rather than acute antimanic response (discussed later in this chapter). Since episode duration is relatively short in rapid cyclers, an episode may end spontaneously before a treatment has had time to become effective. Taylor and Abrams (1981) reported that four or more affective episodes per year did not predict a poor response to treatment of acute mania. It is not clear from their study, however, that the favorable response was actually due to treatment rather than spontaneous remission.

Mixed or dysphoric mania.   It is generally accepted that patients experiencing mixed or dysphoric mania do not respond well to lithium. What remains to be determined is whether they respond better to alternative treatments. Two reviews (Goodwin and Jamison 1990; McElroy and colleagues 1992) emphasized that over the years mixed states have been defined by a variety of criteria (in DSM-IV, a mixed episode must meet criteria for both a major depressive episode and a manic episode every day for at least 1 week). Nonetheless, a consistent observation across most studies is that mixed states are common—40.1% of manic episodes in the study by Goodwin and Jamison (1990) and 31% in the study by McElroy and colleagues (1992)—and that lithium response is poor (roughly half that of nondysphoric or "pure" mania) (Dilsaver et al. 1993a, 1993b; McElroy et al. 1992). McElroy and colleagues (1992) pointed out, however, that "we know of no placebo-controlled studies of lithium in the treatment of acute dysphoric mania" (p. 1638) and that some patients with mixed mania may respond slowly but not less well to lithium. Dilsaver et al. (1993b) suggested that "CBZ [carbamazepine] and VPA [valproate] may be the drugs of choice among the currently available pharmacologic treatments should one opt to treat a patient with dysphoric or mixed mania with one agent alone," yet they acknowledged that adequate comparative trials with lithium have not been performed. In addition, the same group (1993a) described a poorer antimanic response (43%) in 21 patients with mixed mania treated with a variety of antimanic agents including lithium, carbamazepine, and valproate. As the results of the recent lithium-valproate-placebo multicenter trial of acute mania become available, more light may be shed on whether dysphoric mania responds better to valproate than to lithium. At present, it is premature to conclude that there is one preferred monotherapy for mixed mania. It is likely that combination therapies will be the rule.

Age. Age at illness onset and age at time of treatment have not been useful predictors of lithium response in acute mania, although admittedly the issue has not been thoroughly studied. It is difficult to isolate age from confounding variables such as the number of prior episodes, associated medical and psychiatric illnesses, and concomitant medications. A favorable response to lithium is common in the elderly (Young and Klerman 1992), suggesting that age, per se, should not discriminate against a trial of lithium.

Family history. A family history of bipolar disorder has been thought to predict a more favorable antimanic response to lithium, yet there have been no studies to assess this impression. In fact, Taylor and Abrams (1981) found that "the morbidity risk for affective disorder in first-degree relatives failed to differentiate the good from the poor responders" (p. 802). Perhaps it is family history of a positive antimanic response to lithium that predicts a positive response to lithium in a particular patient rather than the history of bipolar disorder itself.

Biological Predictors

Using the laboratory to predict antimanic response to lithium has produced a series of raised, then dashed, expectations. Serry (1969) reported that patients who excreted less lithium after a loading dose of lithium carbonate (lithium retainers) responded better to lithium therapy. Efforts by others to replicate this finding were unsuccessful (summarized in Marini 1980).

Sullivan and colleagues (1977) noted that patients who responded to lithium had higher platelet monoamine oxidase activity than patients who did not respond. Although the design of this study has been criticized (Marini 1980) and the results questioned, attempts have not been made to replicate the findings.

Efforts to correlate urine and cerebrospinal fluid (CSF), neurotransmitter, and metabolite levels with outcome have been unsuccessful (Carroll 1979; Swann et al. 1987). Swann et al. (1987) studied 19 manic patients and found no relationship between outcome and pretreatment levels of CSF homovanillic acid (HVA), 5-hydroxyindoleacetic acid (5-HIAA), and 3-methoxy-4-hydroxyphenylglycol (MHPG), and urinary MHPG, vanillylmandelic acid (VMA), normetanephrine, norepinephrine, and epinephrine. Patients who did and did not respond differed in the fact in that the latter "had higher ratios of urinary MHPG excretion to total synthesis . . . and lower VMA-total synthesis ratios" (p. 439). Even if these findings from a small number of patients could be replicated, they would hardly be of practical value to clinicians.

Red blood cell (RBC) choline levels are increased by lithium therapy, although neither the extent of the increase nor the RBC/plasma choline ratio during treatment reliably predicts response. Stoll and colleagues (1991) measured pretreatment RBC choline levels in 36 acutely manic patients and defined a group with high levels and another with lower levels (similar to controls). They found that the high RBC choline patients were more severely ill, had a worse outcome, required more neuroleptic drug, and, overall, responded less well to lithium. One wonders whether the severity of the mania was the primary response predictor, with high choline levels being an epiphenomenon.

Prophylaxis

Efforts to predict response to long-term maintenance (prophylactic) lithium therapy have been much more extensive than for acute mania or depression. According to Abou-Saleh and Coppen (1990, p. 34), "The most useful predictor of response to prophylactic lithium is, however, an empirical one: a trial of lithium over 6 months to 1 year appears to determine the likelihood of the patient's responding to it in the years to come." For response prediction to be of great clinical value, however, this 6–12-month wait would have to be eliminated and the necessary information provided before or shortly after initiation of treatment. Whether sufficient information is currently available to allow such "up front" prediction is open to question.

Demographic and Clinical Predictors

Grof and colleagues (1983a, 1983b, 1993) conducted a series of studies that examined a number of potentially predictive variables. Factors that had positive predictive value included 1) a primary affective disorder diagnosis, 2) an episodic course with periods of euthymia, 3) absence of rapid cycling, 4) a mania-depression-euthymia episode sequence, 5) a positive family history of bipolar disorder, 6) a normal Minnesota Multiphasic Personality Inventory (MMPI) profile during optimal functioning, 7) the presence of the M antigen in the MNS blood group system, and 8) a greater decrease in prolactin response to hypoglycemia (Grof et al. 1983a). Of particular interest is the fact that the first three clinical variables (diagnosis of affective disorder, episodic course with euthymic intervals, and non-rapid cycling) accounted for most of the predictive power; the other five factors added little. A good response was described as "an episodic illness with prominent affective features, with good quality of free intervals and a low to moderate annual frequency of episodes" (Grof et al. 1983a, p. 198). In a prospective study, their ability to predict response and nonresponse had a "hit rate" of 83% (Grof et al. 1983a).

Aagaard and Vestergaard (1990) evaluated outcome predictors in a prospective two-year study of 133 patients with affective disorders who comprised three groups (bipolar, unipolar, and undetermined). Patients were first divided into nonadherent ($n = 56$) and adherent ($n = 77$) treatment groups. Nonadherence was not predicted by diagnostic subgroup, age, male sex, life events, number of illness-free intervals in the previous 2 years, mood-incongruent psychotic features, or antisocial personality traits. The following were of some predictive value for noncompliance: substance abuse, smoking, young age at onset of illness, and many previous psychiatric hospitalizations. Unfortunately, only 15% of the variance in the prediction analysis of nonadherence could be explained. In patients who were compliant with treatment, predictors of nonresponse included young age, female sex, and a lengthy index episode. Again, diagnostic subgroups were not predictive, nor were recent life events, unfavorable social background, or antisocial personality traits.

Compared with the study by Grof and colleagues, in which affective diagnosis, episode-free interval, and nondeviant personality had important predictive value, the Aagaard and Vestergaard study found that these factors were trends that were not significant. The authors suggested that their patients were more chronic (of 61 bipolar patients, 62% adhered to treatment, and only 32% of the adherent group had no hospitalizations, giving an overall response rate of 12 of 61, or 20%).

Abou-Saleh and Coppen (1990) conducted an open study of 83 unipolar and 31 bipolar patients treated with long-term lithium (range 2–12 years, mean 5.9 years). Overall, bipolar patients responded better than unipolar, but those with "pure familial depressive disorder" did as well as those with bipolar disorder. By combining clinical and personality features, 76% of patients were correctly classified as responders or nonresponders. When response to a 6–12-month trial of lithium was added, the predictive power increased to 96%. In other words, bipolar or endogenous unipolar patients with normal personalities who responded favorably to a 6–12-month trial of lithium were highly likely to do well in the future. Unfortunately, it was the positive prophylactic response to lithium that was the most useful predictor of a longer-term positive prophylactic response to lithium.

Age at illness onset, age at start of lithium, sex, race, nationality, and marital status have shown no useful predictive value (Abou-Saleh 1993; Goodwin and Jamison 1990). It should be noted that lithium maintenance studies have not been done in the elderly (Young and Klerman 1992).

Diagnosis. Since the efficacy of lithium prophylaxis in bipolar disorder has been well established in controlled studies, it stands to reason that a diagnosis of bipolar disorder would predict a favorable response to lithium. But, does bipolar II disorder respond as well as bipolar I? Based on limited data, it probably does, especially if the study design controls for comorbid personality disorder and substance abuse (Abou-Saleh 1993; Goodwin and Jamison 1990).

In terms of schizoaffective disorder, the diagnostic uncertainty that has haunted this "condition" makes definitive statements difficult. Somewhat surprisingly, results of more recent studies suggest lithium efficacy in schizoaffective disorder is equal to that in bipolar disorder (Goodnick and Meltzer 1984; Goodwin and Jamison 1990). Patients with more affective than schizophrenic features and those with more schizomanic than schizodepressive episodes tend to do better.

With regard to the unipolar/bipolar division, the literature tends to support similar prophylactic efficacy for lithium. As summarized in Goodwin and Jamison (1990), unipolar prophylactic studies have been relatively short term and often characterized by more diagnostic heterogeneity than bipolar studies. As noted above, although Abou-Saleh and Coppen (1990) found equal efficacy for lithium in bipolar and pure familial depressive disorder, there was a lesser response in sporadic depressive disorder and depressive spectrum disorder.

Mixed or dysphoric mania. Patients with mixed or dysphoric mania are reputed to respond less well to lithium prophylaxis than patients with pure mania; however, support for this hypothesis is less firm than is generally believed (McElroy et al. 1992). In a 2-year maintenance study, Prien and colleagues (1988) found a poorer response to lithium or lithium plus imipramine in patients with a mixed index episode. Similar findings were described in small open studies by Secunda and colleagues (1985) and Himmelhoch and colleagues (1976). On the other hand, an earlier uncontrolled study found a reasonably good response in patients with mixed episodes followed for 1–5 years (Baastrup and Schou 1967). Overall, available evidence leans toward patients with dysphoric mania having a reduced likelihood of responding well to long-term lithium maintenance. Whether or not lithium alternatives can offer a better long-term prognosis for these patients must be determined.

Rapid cycling. Patients with rapid cycling bipolar disorder (four or more episodes per year) respond less well to lithium prophylaxis than do non-rapid cyclers. As summarized by Post (1990), most but not all studies support this finding. The "inventors" of the concept of rapid cycling found that only 18% of rapid cyclers responded to lithium prophylaxis in contrast to 59% of non-rapid cyclers (Dunner and Fieve 1974). In a retrospective review of 98 patients (including 91 who were bipolar), patients who cycled rapidly before lithium tratment had more depressive symptoms per visit than slower cyclers but showed no statistically significant difference with regard to manic relapses while being treated with lithium (Goodnick et al. 1987). It should be noted that although rapid cyclers as a group respond less well to lithium, many have partial and some have strikingly good responses (Maj 1992). Such a patient is illustrated in Figure 4–1 (Schou 1956). Controlled studies have not been done to determine the relative effectiveness of lithium and its alternatives in rapid cycling, although case reports and open series suggest that carbamazepine and valproate can be beneficial.

Episode frequency.   Response prediction based on the number of previous episodes overlaps to a certain extent with rapid cy-

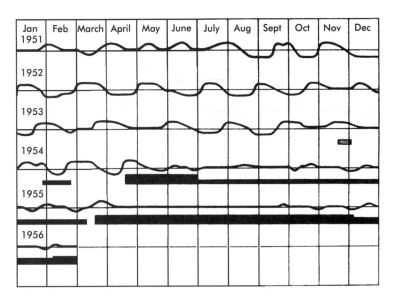

Figure 4–1. The effect of lithium therapy (black bar) on rapid cycling bipolar disorder.
Source.   Reprinted with permission from Schou M: Lithiumterapi ved mani: praktiske retningslinier. *Nord Med* 55:790–794, 1956.

cling. By definition, total episode numbers accrue more rapidly in rapid cyclers. As a result, it may be difficult to separate episode total from episode frequency in terms of the contribution of each to nonresponse. O'Connell et al. (1991) found that the best predictor of poor response to prophylaxis was frequent psychiatric hospitalizations before lithium treatment. In a maintenance therapy study comparing standard versus low serum lithium levels, Gelenberg and colleagues (1989) concluded "that patients with three or more previous mood episodes are not protected by lithium, regardless of the level, although the marginal P value for the interaction effect in our study makes this association insecure" (p. 1492). What is not clear from this and other studies is whether the correlation of high episode frequency and poor response to lithium occurred only in patients who had a prior history of treatment failure, or also in those who were receiving adequate therapy for the first time despite many previous episodes.

The 2-year prospective prophylactic lithium study of Aagaard and Vestergaard (1990) that found poor response rates in patients with many prior hospitalizations did not describe prior treatments for these patients, including whether or not they had previously responded to lithium. Since this Danish study was conducted in the early 1980s, it is likely that at least some patients who did not respond had already demonstrated lithium resistance and that nonresponse was not determined merely by number of previous episodes. For example, the earlier studies of lithium prophylaxis tended to have favorable outcomes despite enrolling patients with numerous prior episodes (Baastrup and Schou 1967).

The following two cases are examples of patients from the author's practice who responded extremely well to lithium despite frequent prior episodes:

1. Between 1959 and 1974, a man with bipolar disorder had 11 hospitalizations totalling 2 years and 5 months. He began lithium prophylaxis in 1974 and has had no further hospitalizations (as of December 1993).
2. A woman, currently age 69, had been hospitalized 10 times for manic or depressive episodes between 1945 and 1978. She was stabilized on lithium prophylaxis and has had no further mood episodes over a 15-year follow-up.

Episode sequence.   The clinical course of bipolar disorder does not always have a consistent pattern of episode sequence, but when it does, the sequence may have some value in predicting response to lithium prophylaxis. Faedda and colleagues (1991) reviewed five studies and found that a mania-depression-euthymia sequence predicted a good response to lithium (a 72% crude response rate), and a depression-mania-euthymia sequence predicted a poor response (a 39% crude response rate). Although all studies that examined the sequence-response pattern found similar results, only one was prospective; consequently, Faedda's group concluded that the sensitivity and specificity of these findings "are too limited . . . to justify withholding treatment" (p. 1239).

Interepisode functioning.   Grof and colleagues (1983a, 1983b, 1993) and Goodnick and colleagues (1987) both found that patients who functioned well between episodes responded best to lithium. Although the latter study was a retrospective evaluation of patients who were already receiving lithium, the former assessed the quality of remission before initiating treatment and also found it to be a strong predictor of a favorable response to lithium.

Index episode.   Does the nature of the index episode (the episode after which prophylactic treatment is initiated) influence the outcome of lithium therapy? Most long-term studies have not considered the effect that the index episode (mania, mixed, or depressed) might have on outcome. Of the studies that examined this, three different results were reported. One study reported that a manic index episode predicted a more favorable response to lithium than a depressive index episode (median time in remission more than 12.6 months versus 3.4 months) (Shapiro et al. 1989); another study reported that a mixed index episode predicted either a poorer outcome (as discussed previously in this chapter) or no relationship (Maj et al. 1985).

Acute response.   The rather obvious question of whether a positive acute response to lithium predicts a favorable prophylactic response does not have an obvious answer. Goodwin and Jamison (1990, pp. 698–699) stated that, "to our knowledge and surprise, there are no systematic studies on the relationship between acute antimanic or antidepressant response to lithium and prophylactic response, although clinical experience suggests that acute response probably does predict prophylactic response." Svestka and Nahunek (1975) found in an open study that acute response predicted prophylactic response and acute nonresponse predicted prophylactic nonresponse. This study supports an acute/prophylactic response relationship, but the limited information provided does not establish the strength of the relationship.

Personality factors. It is generally agreed that severe character pathology predicts a poorer response to lithium prophylaxis of bipolar disorder (it probably predicts a poorer response to any treatment of any condition). Efforts to examine personality variables in response prediction have been inconclusive, in part, because "in virtually all studies, the affective state at the time of personality testing was variable, as were the diagnostic inclusion criteria and measures of treatment success" (Goodwin and Jamison 1990, p. 301). In addition, most studies have examined short-term rather than long-term response to lithium (Abou-Saleh 1993). Also in question is whether personality factors are more predictive of compliance than response (for example, obsessional tendencies were associated with better adherence to treatment) (Abou-Saleh 1993). In general, personality tests have not established themselves as being clinically useful in lithium response prediction.

Family factors. Miklowitz and colleagues (1988) reported that bipolar patients in families with high levels of expressed emotion and negative affective style were at a much increased risk of affective relapse. Because the sample size was small ($N = 33$) and mixed (bipolar and schizoaffective patients), and because only eight patients were on lithium alone, the results must be viewed with caution. The results were supported, however, in a larger long-term outcome study (O'Connell et al. 1991). Further studies of family psychosocial factors as well as other aspects of social support are clearly indicated.

Family history. Maj (1992) critically reviewed the relationship between family history of mood disorder and effectiveness of lithium prophylaxis and noted that most studies found a better outcome in association with a positive family history. In those studies focusing on bipolar disorder, lithium response was 80% when family history was positive compared with 50% when it was negative. A family history of nonbipolar mood disorder does not appear to have predictive value with regard to lithium prophylaxis.

A second family history issue is whether a relative's favorable response to lithium is predictive of a favorable response to lithium in the proband. Such a relationship was supported by the twin study of Mendlewicz (1979) and others, but overall, pharmacogenetic studies of lithium response are not as well defined as one might expect. Nonetheless, it seems reasonable to expect that a positive response to lithium in a *close* relative would predict a positive response in a patient with the same disorder.

Biological Predictors

It is tempting to summarize the quest for biological predictors of effective lithium prophylaxis as futile and let it go at that. However, since the final answer to response prediction probably lies in biology, an update seems in order.

Neuroendocrine factors. The dexamethasone suppression test (DST) has not been shown to be of predictive value (Abou-Saleh 1993). Abnormalities of the hypothalamic-pituitary-thyroid axis have been associated with a poorer response to lithium (Abou-Saleh 1993), and there is some evidence that correcting these abnormalities may restore treatment responsiveness. Abnormal thyroid function, per se, should not be a deterrent to the implementation of long-term treatment with lithium, but obviously the abnormalities may need to be corrected.

RBC/plasma lithium ratio. Intuitively, it makes sense to assume that the inside of RBCs is more similar to the inside of brain cells than is serum or plasma, and that measuring lithium within these cells might be a way to predict treatment outcome. These measurements have been made repeatedly, but have only provoked controversy. Since 1979, considerable research has been done on the RBC/plasma lithium ratio (summarized in Carroll 1979), but no definitive answer has been obtained. Since then, Maj and colleagues (1984) found a statistically significant difference ($P < .01$)

between the ratio in patients who responded (.40 ± .08) and patients who did not respond (.36 ± .05), but the overlap among individuals appears to neutralize any clinical utility the test might
have. Meanwhile, when Grof and colleagues (1993) corrected for
variables affecting the ratio such as age, sex, and plasma lithium
level, "there was no variance left to be explained by the lithium
response" (p. 17). The future of the RBC/plasma lithium ratio as a
predictor of prophylactic lithium response is not promising.

Blood group antigens.   Maj and colleagues (1985) and Perris and
colleagues (1979) reported that a poor prophylactic response to
lithium in bipolar (but not unipolar) patients was predicted by the
presence of the HLA-A3 antigen. Grof and colleagues (1993) investigated the MNS blood group system and found that the presence of the M antigen predicted a favorable response to lithium
(although clinical factors accounted for almost all the variance that
could be explained). Replication of these blood group antigen
findings is necessary before any firm conclusions can be reached.

Other.   Platelet monoamine oxidase activity did not correlate
with response to lithium prophylaxis (Abou-Saleh 1993; Grof et
al. 1983a). Grof and colleagues (1993) found a greater decrease in
prolactin response to hypoglycemia in patients who responded
than in patients who did not respond, and although they described this as a "robust finding" they have been unable to put it
to clinical use. Abou-Saleh (1993) found that serotonin transport
into platelets correlated with long-term outcome; patients with
an increase in V_{max} did better. A variety of other factors have been
reported to predict response to long-term lithium therapy, but
none has been adequately substantiated. These include audi-
tory evoked potentials (Hegerl and Herrmann 1990), rectal mu-
cosal potential difference (summarized in Carroll 1979), RBC
calcium binding (Abou-Saleh 1993), RBC sodium, potassium-
adenosine triphosphatase activity (Goodwin and Jamison 1990),
reduced urinary MHPG level (summarized in Jefferson et al.
1987), and increased serum calcium and magnesium (summarized in Jefferson et al. 1987). In a computed tomography brain
study of bipolar patients, response to lithium treatment did not
correlate with lateral ventricular enlargement (the authors did

not define whether response was due to acute or prophylactic treatment) (Dewan et al. 1988).

Acute Depression

Demographic and Clinical Predictors

A diagnosis of bipolar depression might well be the strongest predictor of a favorable acute antidepressant response to lithium. Goodwin and Jamison (1990) reviewed seven placebo-controlled studies of hospitalized depressed patients and found a positive response to lithium in 79% of patients with bipolar disorder (64 of 81) and only 36% of the unipolar patients (20 of 55). In double-blind comparative studies with tricyclic antidepressants, lithium was generally found to be at least as effective as the tricyclics (in four of five studies), although those studies did not separate unipolar and bipolar depression in terms of treatment response. Zornberg and Pope (1993) pointed out that there have been no placebo-controlled studies comparing the efficacy of lithium and a conventional antidepressant in patients stratified according to bipolar versus unipolar depression.

Some clinicians believe that patients with anergic, hypersomnic, hyperphagic depressions respond more favorably to lithium than patients with anxiety, insomnia, and anorexia, regardless of whether the patients have bipolar or major depressive disorder. This hypothesis remains to be formally tested.

"Personality" predictors of response have never been well established. In 1978, Donnelly and colleagues administered pretreatment MMPIs to unipolar and bipolar depressed patients and, after identifying patients who did and did not respond to lithium, determined the combination of individual items that best predicted outcome. When these items were tested prospectively in a small group of patients, they were reported to be 100% accurate in distinguishing patients who would respond from patients who would not. Another group also reported some predictive value with another variation of the MMPI Clinical Scales (House and Martin 1975). Nothing has been reported about these approaches since the 1970s.

Family history has not been shown to be of predictive value

with regard to the antidepressant effect of lithium (although this observation was based only on one small study).

Biological Predictors

Most of the work that attempted to find biological predictors of an antidepressant response to lithium was performed quite a few years ago and has been summarized by several authors (Carroll 1979; Jefferson et al. 1987; Marini 1980). Studies have examined serum calcium/magnesium ratios, CSF 5-HIAA and urinary MHPG levels, RBC catechol-o-methyltransferase level, platelet monoamine oxidase activity, an augmenting average-evoked response on the electroencephalogram, RBC/plasma lithium ratio, and an activation response to amphetamine challenge. None of these tests seems to be of clinical value and none appears to be in current use for predicting lithium response.

More recently, nuclear magnetic resonance proton T_1 relaxation times were noted to be higher in bipolar depressed patients than in normal control subjects and nonbipolar depressed patients. Patients who responded to lithium (five of six bipolar patients) had a substantial decrease in T_1 relaxation time during treatment (Rosenthal et al. 1986). Whether or not the higher T_1 relaxation times predicted bipolarity as opposed to lithium response could not be determined. Also, this study involved only eight patients. Finally, the use of nuclear magnetic resonance imaging to predict treatment response would hardly be of practical clinical use.

Lithium Augmentation for Resistant Depression

The majority of investigators believe that lithium augmentation is effective in at least 50% of patients with antidepressant-resistant depression. According to de Montigny (1992), "at present, no valid predictor of the likelihood of response to lithium augmentation has been clearly identified" (p. 5). In his comprehensive review, Johnson (1991) was not any more optimistic about predicting response to lithium augmentation, although there was some suggestion that bipolar patients respond better than unipolar. Since unipolar patients also respond reasonably well, however, this finding has no great predictive value.

Conclusion

The best way to predict response to lithium is with an empirical trial of lithium. The second best way to predict response to lithium is by certain clinical characteristics (classic bipolar disorder, few prior episodes, good interepisode functioning, and a mania-depression-euthymia cycle). Biological predictors are of little or no value although, ultimately, clinical response should be best determined by biological testing, much in the same way that sensitivity testing currently determines response to antibiotic treatment. In the future, the laboratory should be able to report, in advance of treatment, whether a patient will or will not respond to lithium. Ideally, the report will also provide similar information about other mood stabilizers so that clinicians may choose the pharmacologic treatment most likely to be effective in a given patient.

References

Aagaard J, Vestergaard P: Predictors of outcome in prophylactic lithium treatment: a 2-year prospective study. J Affect Disord 18:259–266, 1990

Abou-Saleh MT: Who responds to prophylactic lithium therapy? Br J Psychiatry 163(suppl 21):20–26, 1993

Abou-Saleh MT, Coppen AJ: Predictors of long-term outcome of mood disorder on prophylactic lithium. Lithium 1:27–35, 1990

Baastrup PC, Schou M: Lithium as a prophylactic agent: its effect against recurrent depressions and manic-depressive psychosis. Arch Gen Psychiatry 16:162–172, 1967

Carroll BJ: Prediction of treatment outcome with lithium. Arch Gen Psychiatry 36:870–878, 1979

Cohen S, Khan A, Cox G: Demographic and clinical features predictive of recovery in acute mania. J Nerv Ment Dis 177:638–642, 1989

Dewan MJ, Haldipur CV, Boucher MF, et al: Bipolar affective disorder, II: EEG, neuropsychological, and clinical correlates of CT abnormality. Acta Psychiatr Scand 77:677–682, 1988

Dilsaver SC, Swann AC, Shoaib AM, et al: Depressive mania associated with nonresponse to antimanic agents. Am J Psychiatry 150:1548–1551, 1993a

Dilsaver SC, Swann AC, Shoaib AM, et al: The manic syndrome: factors which may predict a patient's response to lithium, carbamazepine and valproate. J Psychiatry Neurosci 18:61–66, 1993b

Donnelly EF, Goodwin FK, Waldman IN, et al: Prediction of antidepressant responses to lithium. Am J Psychiatry 135:552–556, 1978

DuFour H, Pringuey D, Milech T (eds): The Prediction of Lithium Response. Marseille, France, Marseille University, 1983

Dunner DL, Fieve RR: Clinical factors in lithium carbonate prophylaxis failure. Arch Gen Psychiatry 30:229–233, 1974

Faedda GL, Baldessarini RJ, Tohen M, et al: Episode sequence in bipolar disorder and response to lithium treatment. Am J Psychiatry 148:1237–1239, 1991

Gelenberg AJ, Kane JM, Keller MB, et al: Comparison of standard and low serum levels of lithium for maintenance treatment of bipolar disorder. N Engl J Med 321:1489–1493, 1989

Goodnick PJ, Meltzer HY: Treatment of schizoaffective disorders. Schizophr Bull 10:30–48, 1984

Goodnick PJ, Fieve RR, Schlegel A, et al: Predictors of interepisode symptoms and relapse in affective disorder patients treated with lithium carbonate. Am J Psychiatry 144:367–369, 1987

Goodwin FK, Jamison KR: Manic-Depressive Illness. New York, Oxford University Press, 1990

Grof P, Hux M, Grof E, et al: Prediction of response to stabilizing lithium treatment. Pharmacopsychiatria 16:195–200, 1983a

Grof P, Lane J, Hux M, et al: Predicting the response to long-term lithium treatment: interim results of a prospective study, in The Prediction of Lithium Response (Proceedings from symposium in Marseille, France; June 2–3, 1980). Edited by Dufour H, Pringuey D, Milech T. Marseille, France, Marseille University, 1983b, pp 43–53

Grof P, Alda M, Grof E, et al: The challenge of predicting response to stabilizing lithium treatment. The importance of patient selection. Br J Psychiatry 163(suppl 21):16–19, 1993

Hegerl U, Herrmann WM: Event-related potentials and the prediction of differential drug response in psychiatry. Neuropsychobiology 23:99–108, 1990

Himmelhoch JM, Mulla D, Neil JF, et al: Incidence and significance of mixed affective states in a bipolar population. Arch Gen Psychiatry 33:1062–1066, 1976

House KM, Martin RL: MMPI delineation of a subgroup of depressed patients refractory to lithium carbonate therapy. Am J Psychiatry 132:644–646, 1975

Jefferson JW, Greist JH, Ackerman DL, et al: Lithium encyclopedia for clinical practice, 2nd Edition. Washington, DC, American Psychiatric Press, 1987, pp 565–574

Johnson FN: Lithium augmentation therapy for depression. Reviews in Contemporary Pharmacotherapy 2:1–52, 1991

Maj M: Clinical prediction of response to lithium prophylaxis in bipolar patients: a critical update. Lithium 3:15–21, 1992

Maj M, Del Vecchio M, Starace F, et al: Prediction of affective psychoses response to lithium prophylaxis: the role of socio-demographic, clinical, psychological and biological variables. Acta Psychiatr Scand 69:37–44, 1984

Maj M, Arena F, Lovero N, et al: Factors associated with response to lithium prophylaxis in DSM-III major depression and bipolar disorder. Pharmacopsychiatry 18:309–313, 1985

Marini JL: Predicting lithium responders and nonresponders: physiological indicators, in Handbook of Lithium Therapy. Edited by Johnson FN. Lancaster, England, MTP Press, 1980, pp 118–125

McElroy SL, Keck PE Jr, Pope HG, et al: Clinical and research implications of the diagnosis of dysphoric or mixed mania or hypomania. Am J Psychiatry 149:1633–1644, 1992

Mendlewicz J: Prediction of treatment outcome: family and twin studies in lithium prophylaxis and the question of lithium red blood cell/plasma ratios, in Lithium: Controversies and Unresolved Issues. Edited by Cooper TB, Gershon S, Kline NS, Schou M. Amsterdam, Exerpta Medica, 1979, pp 226–240

Miklowitz DJ, Goldstein MJ, Nuechterlein KH, et al: Family factors and the course of bipolar affective disorder. Arch Gen Psychiatry 45:225–231, 1988

Miller F, Tanebaum JH, Griffin A, et al: Prediction of treatment response in bipolar, manic disorder. J Affect Disord 21:75–78, 1991

de Montigny C: Lithium augmentation in refractory depression. Canadian Review of Affective Disorders 2(4):3–6, 1992

Murphy DL, Beigel A: Depression, elation, and lithium carbonate responses in manic patient subgroups. Arch Gen Psychiatry 31:643–648, 1974

O'Connell RA, Mayo JA, Flatow L, et al: Outcome of bipolar disorder on long-term treatment with lithium. Br J Psychiatry 159:123–129, 1991

Perris C, Strandman E, Wählby: HL-A antigens and the response to prophylactic lithium. Neuropsychobiology 5:114–118, 1979

Post RM: Prophylaxis of bipolar affective disorders. Int Rev Psychiatr 2 (3–4):277–320, 1990

Prien RF, Kupfer DJ, Mansky PA, et al: Drug therapy in the prevention of recurrences in unipolar and bipolar affective disorders. Arch Gen Psychiatry 41:1096–1104, 1984

Prien RF, Himmelhoch JM, Kupfer DJ: Treatment of mixed mania. J Affect Disord 15:9–15, 1988

Rosenthal J, Strauss A, Minkoff L, et al: Identifying lithium-responsive bipolar depressed patients using nuclear magnetic resonance. Am J Psychiatry 143:779–780, 1986

Schou M: Lithiumterapi ved mani: praktiske retningslinier. Nord Med 55:790–794, 1956

Secunda SK, Katz MM, Swann A, et al: Mania: diagnosis, state measurement and prediction of treatment response. J Affect Disord 8:113–121, 1985

Serry M: The lithium excretion test, I: clinical applications and interpretation. Aust N Z J Psychiatry 3:390–394, 1969

Shapiro DR, Quitkin FM, Fleiss JL: Response to maintenance therapy in bipolar illness: effect of index episode. Arch Gen Psychiatry 46:401–405, 1989

Stokes PE, Stoll PM, Shamoian CA, et al: Efficacy of lithium as acute treatment of manic-depressive illness. Lancet 1:1319–1325, 1971

Sullivan JL, Cavenar JO, Maltbie A, et al: Platelet-monoamine-oxidase activity predicts response to lithium in manic-depressive illness. Lancet 2:1325–1327, 1977

Svestka J, Nahunek K: The result of lithium therapy in acute phases of affective psychoses and some other prognostical factors of lithium prophylaxis. Act Nerv Super (Praha) 17:270–271, 1975

Swann AC, Secunda SK, Katz MM, et al: Lithium treatment of mania: clinical characteristics, specificity of symptom change, and outcome. Psychiatry Res 18:127–141, 1986

Swann AC, Koslow SH, Katz MM, et al: Lithium carbonate treatment of mania: cerebrospinal fluid and urinary monoamine metabolites and treatment outcome. Arch Gen Psychiatry 44:345–354, 1987

Taylor MA, Abrams R: Prediction of treatment response in mania. Arch Gen Psychiatry 38:800–803, 1981

Young RC, Klerman GL: Mania in late life: focus on age at onset. Am J Psychiatry 149:867–876, 1992

Zornberg GL, Pope HG: Treatment of depression in bipolar disorder: new directions for research. J Clin Psychopharmacol 13:397–408, 1993

CHAPTER 5

Carbamazepine in Bipolar Disorder

Charles L. Bowden, M.D.

Carbamazepine was first reported as useful in treating bipolar disorder by Takezaki and Hanaoka in 1971. Since that time, reports involving more than 800 patients have been published; therefore, an extensive experience with carbamazepine is available. In the aggregate, the studies have substantial limitations. Many did not define their subjects well. Few were double-blind, and several of those were not randomized. Only one acute study of 19 patients compared carbamazepine to placebo, and the varying duration of treatment and A-B-A (off-on-off) design limit the conclusions to be drawn (Post et al. 1987). The majority of controlled studies did not utilize carbamazepine as monotherapy; therefore, many of the results do not establish whether carbamazepine alone, with another concurrently administered drug, or the combined effect of the two drugs accounted for the results obtained. Additionally, no multicenter trials of carbamazepine have been published, thus the possibility cannot be ruled out that the results obtained were not influenced by biasing factors tied to the particular center. Given these caveats, we have assumed that if two or more studies by unrelated investigative groups report consistent results, the relationship is a probable one; similarly, relationships reported only once, or with mixed results across studies, will be viewed as possible.

The issue of prediction of treatment response can be addressed at several levels. The first step is assessing the information that the psychiatrist may have available before implementation of treatment. This includes prior response to treatments, current symptomatology, current severity, prior illness course, family history of mental illness, and ancillary laboratory or special procedure information. Additionally, information that may develop during treatment can also be viewed as predictive of outcome. Examples include plasma concentrations of drug, changes in biochemical parameters, early symptomatic change, which is associated with subsequent recovery or nonrecovery, and evidence of efficacy or lack of efficacy with concurrently administered medications, which will be addressed in turn, although in some categories no published information is available.

Factors Associated with Acute Treatment Response

Response to Prior Treatments

Studies published since the mid-1980s indicate that at least 40% of patients either do not respond well to lithium, or if they respond, they are unable to tolerate its side effects at therapeutic doses (Potter and Bowden 1992). Although most of these are open, empirical studies, one was a prospective, randomized double-blind comparison in acutely manic patients, which reported that only 33% of patients had moderate or better outcomes after 8 weeks of treatment with lithium (Small et al. 1991). A substantial percentage of patients studied with carbamazepine have not been responsive to previous lithium treatment. Indeed, some of the differences between response rates to carbamazepine in acute treatment studies may be accounted for by studies that have enrolled relatively more patients who do not respond to lithium (Post et al. 1987) and subsequently reported more favorable results than studies with fewer refractory patients (Lerer et al. 1987). A recent study found that among acutely manic patients previously treated with lithium, patients with a previous favorable response did well with lithium treatment in a randomized, double-blind trial, whereas patients who had fared poorly with their most recent treatment showed negligible improvement in the prospective trial (Bowden et al. 1993). Given the substantial evidence from both controlled and uncontrolled trials that carbamazepine is effective in 50%–60% of acutely manic patients (see Table 5–1), perhaps the strongest indication for consideration of carbamazepine therapy is the acutely manic patient who has been unresponsive to an adequate trial of lithium, or unable to tolerate its side effects, and who has no contraindications to a trial of carbamazepine.

Acute Mania

The largest experience with carbamazepine is in the treatment of acute mania (Table 5–1). Controlled studies not confounded by neuroleptic medication report moderate or better response in 29%–66% of patients, with a mean of 58% across studies. These results are comparable to those reported for lithium and valproate (Goodwin and Jamison 1990). In studies that have compared carbamazepine to lithium, two studies reported that the drugs were comparably effective (Okuma et al. 1990; Small et al. 1991), and one reported lithium as more effective than carbamazepine (Lerer et al. 1987). Carbamazepine and neuroleptics were equally effective in three studies (Brown et al. 1989; Grossi et al. 1984; Okuma et al. 1979). By contrast, lithium was superior to neuroleptics in nearly all studies (Goodwin and Jamison 1990). Several studies that have compared carbamazepine plus a neuroleptic to a neuroleptic alone have also indicated a positive additive effect

Table 5–1. Controlled studies of carbamazepine in acute mania

Study	Comparison response	CBZ response	Comparison
Okuma et al. 1979	CPZ	21/31	15/28
Lerer et al. 1987	Li	4/14	11/14
Post et al. 1987	Placebo	12/19	N/A
Okuma et al. 1990	Li[a]	31/50	30/51
Small et al. 1991	Li	8/24	8/24
Totals		**76/138 (55%)**	**64/117 (55%)**

Note.   CBZ = carbamazepine; CPZ = chlorpromazine; Li = lithium; response = moderate or better improvement.
[a]neuroleptics allowed.

(Klein et al. 1984; Muller and Stoll 1984). Additionally most studies that compared carbamazepine with lithium allowed substantial neuroleptic use (Lenzi et al. 1986; Lusznat et al. 1988; Okuma et al. 1990), as did several of the so-called carbamazepine versus placebo or neuroleptic comparison studies (Klein et al. 1984; Muller and Stoll 1984; Takezaki and Hanaoka 1971). Taken in the aggregate, these studies suggest that carbamazepine may be more effective for acute mania when combined with neuroleptics (or lithium) than as monotherapy.

Bipolar Depression

Bipolar depressed patients have shown relatively low rates of response to carbamazepine in one controlled trial (Post et al. 1986) and in case reports (Schaffer et al. 1985). Given that carbamazepine often causes antithyroid activity, it is of interest that the degree of thyroxine reduction was associated with antidepressant responsiveness to carbamazepine (Post et al. 1986); however, it is important to distinguish between acute antidepressant effects of a mood stabilizer and its ability to prevent depressive relapses. No studies have adequately addressed the relative frequency or severity of depressive episodes in bipolar patients treated prophylactically with carbamazepine.

Mixed Mania

Post and colleagues (1989) reported that acutely manic patients who responded better to carbamazepine had higher baseline ratings for depression. In contrast, Lusznat and colleagues (1988) reported that euphoric/grandiose patients did better than patients with irritable/delusional symptomatology, which may be analogous to mixed states. This possible advantage in mixed mania is of importance given the conclusive evidence that lithium is not highly effective in mixed mania (Post et al. 1987; Prien et al. 1988; Secunda et al. 1985). The definition of mixed mania remains somewhat unsettled (McElroy et al. 1992). The proposal of McElroy and colleagues is generally consistent with the DSM-IV requirement for mixed mania of symptoms of a major depressive episode except for the durational requirement (American Psychiatric Association 1994).

Rapid Cycling

Patients with rapid-cycling forms of bipolar disorder may respond better to carbamazepine (Post et al. 1987). Other reports indicate that patients who experienced rapid cycling did less well with carbamazepine treatment than did patients who did not experience rapid cycling (Dilsaver et al. 1993; Joyce 1988). Part of the divergent results may result from lack of clarity regarding the definition of rapid cycling. The current convention is to categorize as rapid cycling any patient who has had four or more episodes of depression, mania, or a combination thereof during the preceding 12 months. It is possible that the number of manic episodes is more associated with poor response than is the number of depressive episodes. Furthermore, rapid-cycling illness course may be a consequence of recent or concurrent antidepressant use, and published reports of rapid-cycling patients have not always characterized patients with regard to this variable. Finally, there is evidence that rapid cycling may characterize illness that has been present for many years as worsening with longer duration of illness (Calabrese et al. 1992). In part because of the difficulties in establishing a definition free of confounds, the approach taken in DSM-IV is to utilize rapid cycling as an illness course modifier rather than a subtype or alternate form per se (American Psychiatric Association 1994). Although the data for carbamazepine remain unsettled, it is clear that rapid cycling is associated with a poor response to lithium (Dunner and Fieve 1974; Goodnick et al. 1987).

Severity

Small and colleagues (1991) reported that patients with greater initial severity did worse with carbamazepine treatment than those with milder symptomatology. In the same study, Small's group reported that psychosis was a negative predictor of response; however, there is substantial overlap between psychosis and overall severity; thus it remains unclear whether both variables are independent predictors. Others have suggested that greater severity is a positive predictor of carbamazepine response (Post et al. 1987).

Secondary Mania

The group of secondary manic disorders—disorders in which a wide range of medical conditions that affect brain structure, function or metabolism may also lead to a generally irritable, mixed manic state —has expanded with better recognition of such manic syndromes (Himmelhoch and Garfinkel 1986; Krauthammer and Klerman 1978). Open studies suggest a better response to carbamazepine than to lithium (Himmelhoch and Garfinkel 1986).

Family History

Ballenger and Post (1980) reported that negative family history for mood disorder was associated with a favorable response to carbamazepine.

Prophylaxis

Five controlled trials studied carbamazepine for prophylaxis. Of the four that compared carbamazepine with lithium, three found no significant differences (Coxhead et al. 1992; Lusznat et al. 1988; Small et al. 1991) and generally reported better tolerance to carbamazepine. The time in remission was greater among lithium-treated than carbamazepine-treated patients (9.3 versus 3.3 months) in another study (Watkins et al. 1987). The one study comparing carbamazepine with placebo found a significant trend for better response with carbamazepine (Okuma et al. 1981).

Additionally, open reports suggest that a substantial number of patients who initially respond well to carbamazepine lose the benefit over time. Frankenberg and colleagues (1988) reported that only eight of 34 patients initially responsive to carbamazepine were still taking it after 3–4 years of maintenance therapy. A pattern of possible treatment-induced refractoriness to carbamazepine has also been described (Post et al. 1990). The number of bipolar patients studied for prophylactic effects of carbamazepine is inadequate to establish any firm conclusions. Because of the methodological difficulties of long-term studies of bipolar disorder, maintenance treatment studies are even more difficult than those for acute treatment; therefore, the situation is not likely to be soon remedied. Nevertheless, given the strong lines of evidence for the value of sustained prophylactic treatment in bipolar disorder, some guidelines for the prophylactic use of carbamazepine are needed by the treating psychiatrist. The author recommends continuation of carbamazepine in patients who responded well to acute-episode treatment. Dosage should be that which maintains approximately the same plasma concentration associated with improvement from the acute manic episode. Since carbamazepine induces its own hepatic metabolism, a compensatory increase in dosage will generally be necessary during the first several months of treatment. Given the evidence that carbamazepine's prophylactic effectiveness may be lost over time, the psychiatrist should be alert to early signs of relapse and promptly alter the treatment regimen, either through dosage adjustment or addition of or change to lithium or valproate.

Potentially Useful Variables

Plasma Levels of Carbamazepine

Because plasma levels are readily obtainable for carbamazepine, and a sigmoid-type concentration-response curve plausibly exists for most drugs, it is surprising that so little data exist in this area; however, studies of plasma drug levels are difficult to conduct outside a hospital setting because of the inability to fully control timing and certainty of drug ingestion as well as timing of blood sampling in relationship to the previous dose. Post and colleagues (1984) found no relationship between plasma level of the epoxide metabolite and response. Empirical evidence suggests that levels of 4 µg/ml or greater are required for response. At the least, we can recommend that a patient not be considered unresponsive unless the steady state plasma level is maintained above 4 µg/ml. Given the enzyme-activating properties of carbamazepine, a dosing increment to overcome the effects of autoinduction will nearly always be needed during the first 2–4 months of treatment.

Combined Therapy

The majority of carbamazepine studies have been of combined therapy, not monotherapy conditions. The concurrent medications have included neuroleptics, lithium, valproate, and combinations thereof (Ketter et al. 1992; Kramlinger and Post 1989). It is likely that better outcomes are achieved for the majority of bipolar patients through use of rationally established combinations of drug therapy than through monotherapy.

Biological Measures

One of the several biological effects of carbamazepine is the reduction of norepinephrine turnover (Waldmeier et al. 1984). Carbamazepine also inhibits stimulation-induced norepinephrine release (Purdy et al. 1977). Carbamazepine has also been shown to reduce norepinephrine in cerebrospinal fluid in four of five manic patients (Post et al. 1985). It would be of interest to know whether carbamazepine-induced norepinephrine reduction is related to improvement in mania, or to the mania's mechanism of action in bipolar disorder.

Implications

In this review we suggest several probable and possible predictors of carbamazepine's effectiveness in bipolar disorder. Since these variables are generally recognizable by a skilled psychiatrist, they are worth utilizing in clinical practice, despite recognition that no single variable has been unequivocally demonstrated as predictive of response or nonresponse to carbamazepine. The strongest recommendations are 1) consideration of carbamazepine for patients who have been unresponsive or intolerant to lithium, and 2) recognition that carbamazepine's role may generally be for combined drug therapy, rather than as monotherapy. Although more specific symptomatic and illness course features may be predictive of or associated with carbamazepine response, their clinical utility in treatment selection may be relatively low.

> *Case 1: Carbamazepine treatment in bipolar disorder.*   A 20-year-old single man, was admitted with the chief complaint from his parents that he was unable to sleep. He had three discrete manic episodes during the previous 2 years, with initial partial control with standard lithium therapy became less effective with each episode. The manic episodes were followed by relatively abrupt

shifts to either mild or severe depressive episodes characterized by psychomotor retardation, brooding, and social withdrawal. His symptoms at the time of admission included elation, agitation, intrusiveness, a threatening manner (including actual blows to staff members on several occasions), thoughts and speech so speeded that conversation was at times impossible, and a severely diminished need for sleep. He believed he was to become the youngest governor of the state and eventually be recognized as a leader of the world by other nations. Most nights during the week before hospitalization he obtained less than 2 hours of sleep. His lithium dose was increased from 1,200 mg before admission to 2,700 mg/day over the first week in hospital. Trifluoperazine was prescribed in an effort to control agitation, hostility, and psychotic thought process as needed initially, then on a scheduled dose of up to 60 mg/day. No sustained improvement resulted from this combined therapy. Due to concern for the safety of staff and other patients, and for the patient, who was unable to provide self-care or eat adequately, he was evaluated for electroconvulsive therapy (ECT). After a series of 16 bilateral ECT treatments, he was moderately improved, with tractable behavior and near-normal psychomotor activity. All lithium medications and the ECT were tolerated well. The patient showed no further improvement and was transferred to an intermediate-term psychiatric hospital.

Treatment at the second hospital consisted of 2,100 mg/day of lithium and trifluoperazine in doses ranging from 15 to 45 mg/day. The patient experienced a return of grandiose delusional symptoms shortly after all efforts to further reduce the neuroleptic. He developed moderately severe extrapyramidal side effects, with drooling, stiffness, occasional dystonic symptomatology, and interference with his usual good psychomotor coordination. Benztropine was effective in relieving the extrapyramidal symptoms, but doses of 12–15 mg/day were required for adequate benefit. He was able to engage in supportive, reality-oriented psychotherapy with his psychiatrist, and in intensive social-milieu therapy at the hospital. After 4 months of treatment, he was transferred to a boarding home and continued in an intensive day-hospital program. A series of relatively ordinary stressors (arguments with parents, his realistic sense that his mother expected more of him than he was capable, failed efforts to date several women, partial impairment of function when he returned to the family business and endeavored to work in the warehouse and product distribution section of their store) contributed to both depressive and manic relapses. Throughout this 3-year period, the patient retained a center of hope, and encouraged his psychiatrist to try alternative therapies.

At several points in treatment, efforts were made to add antidepressants. Often the patient would terminate the medication within the first 2 weeks, claiming that his moods became increasingly unstable. During one relatively severe depressive episode, bupropion was taken and provided apparent improvement in mood within 3 weeks. He felt increasingly agitated after alleviation of the depression and discontinued the bupropion. Valproate was added to the lithium regimen, but was discontinued by the patient after 3 days, when he complained of agitation. Carbamazepine was added with some improvement in sleep, but with development of hypersomnia and subjective complaints that his intellectual state was not optimal for his work efforts. The carbamazepine was discontinued and a trial of clozapine was begun. After an appropriate evaluation, clozapine was added at an initial dosage of 50 mg/day, with a gradual increase to 150 mg/day over a 1-month period, during which time the trifluoperazine therapy was gradually discontinued. The patient reported improvement in mood stability and ability to concentrate, and began speaking about returning to college, despite several abortive efforts to take courses since the onset of his illness.

His social function improved, with the start of a relationship with a woman that lasted for over 6 months. Adverse effects to the clozapine gradually worsened, with drooling, obtundation, frank falling asleep while in conversation with others, and ataxia. The clozapine dosage was reduced to 50 mg/day, but the symptoms of racing thoughts and morbid preoccupation about his illness returned. An increase to 100 mg/day resulted in return of the adverse effects, which were so severe that family members telephoned out of concern that he was endangering himself. The clozapine was discontinued and trifluoperazine restarted. In an effort to better control the returned irritability and mood instability, carbamazepine was restarted, with a dose of 800 mg/day providing a level of around 10 μg/ml. Lithium, estazolam, trifluoperazine, and benztropine were continued. He reported a prompt improvement in his daily mood shifts, less anger, improvement in concentration, and also described himself as better able to handle day-to-day stressors. He appeared to have a fuller range of emotional tone during evaluation.

The patient's social function again improved; however, he remained only marginally functional at work. No additional adverse effects occurred during the next year. Eight months after restarting the carbamazepine, he began to experience more abrupt mood shifts, and became worried about his perceived deterioration in function. He had reliably taken all of his medications and had a stable level of carbamazepine. Efforts to try both a higher and lower carbamazepine dose were without benefit, and the higher dosage was associated with psychomotor obtundation. The carbamazepine was discontinued with alleviation of the adverse effects and no further intensification of symptoms. Two months later he discussed a repeat trial of valproate, which was added and resulted in a partial improvement in symptoms.

This case exemplifies several characteristics of long-term treatment of patients with bipolar disorder. The severe, functionally disabling nature of the illness is apparent. The persistence of delusional thinking without concurrent neuroleptic raises the possibility of a schizoaffective disorder. The patient developed a more rapid cycling form of the disorder over time, with daily mood shifts sometimes present after several years, even during periods in which no antidepressants were taken. Assessment of treatment efficacy was at times complicated by his failure to continue a trial of medication for an adequate period of time. A medication such as carbamazepine, which was initially unsuccessful, may prove beneficial when initiated later in the course of treatment. The high severity of the patient's symptoms did not preclude a substantial benefit from carbamazepine when added to an existing regimen. Over time the patient lost some of the initial benefit associated with the carbamazepine, but difficulties in separating the effects of medications from the subjective impression of the patient could justify a subsequent repeat trial with the carbamazepine.

Conclusion

The extensive but often inconclusive clinical research data support the use of carbamazepine in treatment of bipolar disorder, primarily manic bipolar disorder. Although conclusive findings regarding predictors of treatment response and its associated features are limited, the available information can be combined with other general clinical information about the status of the patient and used as a guide to treatment selection and implementation. Although specific predictive variables are not reliably established, both controlled and open empirical evidence supports the use of carbamazepine, particularly in combination with another mood-stabilizing agent in patients who are refractory to treatment with lithium.

References

American Psychiatric Association: Diagnostic and Statistical Manual of Mental Disorders, 4th Edition. Washington, DC, American Psychiatric Association, 1994

Ballenger JC, Post RM: Carbamazepine in manic-depressive illness: a new treatment. Am J Psychiatry 137:782–790, 1980

Bowden CL, Brugger A, Petty F, et al: Efficacy of valproate in acute mania (abstract). Presented at the annual meeting of the American Psychiatric Association, Washington, DC, May 1993

Brown D, Silverstone T, Cookson J: Carbamazepine compared to haloperidol in acute mania. Int Clin Psychopharmacol 4:229–238, 1989

Calabrese JR, Markovitz PJ, Kimmel SE, et al: Spectrum of efficacy of valproate in 78 rapid-cycling manic depressives. J Clin Psychopharmacol (suppl 12):53–56, 1992

Coxhead N, Silverstone T, Cookson J: Carbamazepine versus lithium in the prophylaxis of bipolar affective disorder. Acta Psychiatr Scand 85:114–118, 1992

Dilsaver SC, Swann AC, Shoaib AM, et al: The manic syndrome: factors which may predict a patient's response to lithium, carbamazepine and valproate. J Psychiatry Neuroscience 18:61–66, 1993

Dunner DL, Fieve RR: Clinical factors in lithium carbonate prophylaxis failure. Arch Gen Psychiatry 30:229–233, 1974

Frankenberg FR, Tohen M, Cohen BM, et al: Long term response to carbamazepine: a retrospective study. J Clin Psychopharmacol 8:130–132, 1988

Goodnick PJ, Fieve RR, Schlegel A, et al: Predictors of interepisode symptoms and relapse in affective disorder patients treated with lithium carbonate. Am J Psychiatry 144:367–369, 1987

Goodwin FK, Jamison KR: Manic-Depressive Illness. New York, Oxford University Press, 1990

Grossi E, Sacchetti E, Vita A, et al: Carbamazepine versus chlorpromazine in mania: a double-blind trial, in Anticonvulsants in Affective Disorders. Edited by Emrich HM, Okuma T, Muller AA. Amsterdam, Exerpta Medica, 1984, pp 177–187

Himmelhoch JA, Garfinkel ME: Sources of lithium resistance in mixed mania. Psychopharmacol Bull 22:613–620, 1986

Joyce PR: Carbamazepine in rapid cycling bipolar affective disorder. Int Clin Psychopharmacol 3:123–129, 1988

Ketter TA, Pazzaglia PJ, Post RM: Synergy of carbamazepine and valproic acid in affective illness: case report and review of the literature. J Clin Psychopharmacol 12:276–281, 1992

Klein E, Bental E, Lerer B, et al: Carbamazepine and haloperidol versus placebo and haloperidol in excited psychoses. Arch Gen Psychiatry 41:165–170, 1984

Kramlinger KG, Post RM: Adding lithium carbonate to carbamazepine: antimanic efficacy in treatment-resistant mania. Acta Psychiatr Scand 79:378–385, 1989

Krauthammer C, Klerman GL: Secondary mania: manic syndromes associated with antecedent physical illness or drugs. Arch Gen Psychiatry 35:1333–1339, 1978

Lenzi A, Grossi E, Massimetti G, et al: Use of carbamazepine in acute psychosis: a controlled study. J Int Med Res 14:78–84, 1986

Lerer B, Moore N, Meyendorff E, et al: Carbamazepine versus lithium in mania: a double-blind study. J Clin Psychiatry 48:89–93, 1987

Lusznat RM, Murphy DP, Nunn CMH: Carbamazepine versus lithium in the treatment and prophylaxis of mania. Br J Psychiatry 153:198–204, 1988

McElroy SL, Keck PE Jr, Pope HG, et al: Clinical and research implications of the diagnosis of dysphoric or mixed mania or hypomania. Am J Psychiatry 149:1633–1644, 1992

Muller AA, Stoll KD: Carbamazepine and oxycarbazepine in the treatment of manic syndromes: studies in Germany, in Anticonvulsants in Affective Disorders. Edited by Emirch M, Okuma T, Muller AA. Amsterdam, Excerpta Medica, 1984

Okuma T, Inanaga K, Otsuki S, et al: Comparison of the anti-manic efficacy of carbamazepine and chlorpromazine: a double-blind, controlled study. Psychopharmacology 66:211–217, 1979

Okuma T, Inanaga K, Otsuki S, Sarai K, et al: A preliminary double-blind study of the efficacy of carbamazepine in prophylaxis of manic-depressive illness. Psychopharmacology 73:95–96, 1981

Okuma T, Yamashita L, Takahashi R, et al: Comparison of the antimanic efficacy of carbamazepine and lithium carbonate by double-blind controlled study. Pharmacopsychiatry 23:143–150, 1990

Post RM, Uhde TW, Wofe EA: Profile of clinical efficacy and side effects of carbamazepine in psychiatry illness: relationship to blood and CSF levels of carbamazepine and its -10, 11-epoxide metabolite. Acta Psychiatr Scand (suppl 313):104–120, 1984.

Post RM, Rubinow DR, Uhde TW, et al: Effects of carbamazepine on noradrenergic mechanisms in affectively ill patients. Psychopharmacology 87:59–63, 1985

Post RM, Uhde TW, Roy-Byrne PP, et al: Antidepressant effects of carbamazepine. Am J Psychiatry 143:29–34, 1986

Post RM, Uhde TW, Roy-Byrne PP, et al: Correlates of antimanic response to carbamazepine. Psychiatry Res 21:71–83, 1987

Post RM, Rubinow DR, Uhde TW, et al: Dysphoric mania: clinical and biological correlates. Arch Gen Psychiatry 46:353–358, 1989

Post RM, Leverich G, Rosoff AS et al: Carbamazepine prophylaxis in refractory affective disorders: a focus on long-term follow-up. J Clin Psychopharmacol 10:318–327, 1990

Potter WZ, Bowden CL: Introduction: valproate and mood disorders. Perspectives. J Clin Psychopharmacol 12:52–56, 1992

Prien RF, Himmelhoch JM, Kupfer DJ: Treatment of mixed mania. J Affect Disord 15:9–15, 1988

Purdy RE, Julien RM, Fairhurst AS, et al: Effect of carbamazepine on the in vitro uptake and release of norepinephrine in adrenergic nerves of rabbit aorta and in whole brain synaptosome. Epilepsia 18:251–257, 1977

Secunda S, Katz M, Swann A, et al: Mania: diagnosis, state measurement, and prediction of treatment response. J Affect Disord 8:113–121, 1985

Schaffer CB, Mungas D, Rockwell E: Successful treatment of psychotic depression with carbamazepine. J Clin Psychopharmacol 5:233–235, 1985

Small JG, Klapper MH, Milstein V, et al: Carbamazepine compared with lithium in the treatment of mania. Arch Gen Psychiatry 48:915–921, 1991

Takezaki H, Hanaoka M: The use of carbamazepine (Tegretol) in the control of manic depressive psychosis and other manic, depressive states. Seishin Shinkeigaku Zasshi 13:173–183, 1971

Waldmeier PC, Baumann PA, Fehr B, et al: Carbamazepine decreases catecholamine turnover in the rat brain. J Pharmacol Exp Ther 231:166–172, 1984

Watkins SE, Callender K, Thomas DR, et al: The effects of carbamazepine and lithium on remission from affective illness. Br J Psychiatry 150:180–182, 1987

CHAPTER 6

Valproate

Scott A. West, M.D., Susan L. McElroy, M.D., and
Paul E. Keck, Jr., M.D.

Valproic acid, a simple branched-chain fatty acid, has been used extensively in the United States in the treatment of epilepsy. It was first recognized as a mood stabilizer in 1966 by Lambert and colleagues, just three years after its anticonvulsant properties were discovered (Keck, Jr. et al. 1993b; Penry and Dean 1989). Valproate is presently available in several preparations: valproic acid (Depakene); sodium valproate (Depakene syrup); divalproex sodium (Depakote), an enteric-coated compound containing valproic acid and sodium valproate in equimolar concentrations; and divalproex sodium sprinkle capsules (Depakote Sprinkle Capsules), which can be pulled apart and sprinkled on food. The term *valproate* will be used to denote all of these formulations.

Since the initial report by Lambert and colleagues (1966), numerous uncontrolled and controlled studies have repeatedly demonstrated the efficacy of valproate in the treatment of bipolar disorder and schizoaffective disorder (McElroy and Keck, Jr. 1993a). Valproate has been studied most extensively in the treatment of acute mania, with over 16 open studies suggesting that valproate may be effective in up to two-thirds of manic patients with bipolar disorder or schizoaffective disorder. Three placebo-controlled studies (Brennan et al. 1984; Emrich et al. 1985; Pope et al. 1991) and one lithium-controlled study (Freeman et al. 1992) have demonstrated that valproate is significantly more effective than placebo and comparable to lithium in the treatment of acute mania in patients with bipolar disorder. Conversely, there are only four uncontrolled reports and no controlled studies of valproate in the treatment of acute unipolar, bipolar, or schizoaffective depression (Calabrese and Delucchi 1990; Hayes 1989; Lambert 1984; McElroy et al. 1988c). Three of these studies suggest that valproate is more effective as an antimanic (62% overall response rate) than an antidepressant agent (30% overall response rate); however, preliminary results from a prospectively followed cohort of patients with rapid-cycling bipolar disorder suggest that valproate may be more effective as an antidepressant when administered over longer periods of time, and that its prophylactic antidepressant effects may be superior to its acute antidepressant effects (Calabrese and Delucchi 1990; Calabrese et al. 1992, 1993b).

Although there have been no controlled clinical trials evaluating the efficacy of valproate in the long-term treatment of bipolar or schizoaffective disorder, open studies suggest that valproate has long-term mood stabilizing effects. Valproate has been reported to decrease the frequency and intensity of recurrent manic and depressive episodes in many patients, including those with rapid cycling, mixed bipolar disorder, bipolar II disorder, and schizoaffective disorder (McElroy et al. 1992).

In this chapter we review a number of factors that are reported to be associated with a therapeutic response to valproate including diagnosis-related factors, clinical course variables, comorbid psychiatric diagnoses, associated neurological factors, family history, and treatment-related variables (see Tables 6–1 and 6–2). Because valproate has been extensively studied in the treatment of mania, predictors of antimanic response will be emphasized, but because data are now becoming available regarding the antidepressant efficacy of valproate, potential predictors of antidepressant response to valproate will also be reviewed.

Potential Predictors of Antimanic Response

Diagnosis-Related Factors

Several studies suggest that patients with a diagnosis of bipolar disorder respond more favorably to valproate than patients with

Table 6–1. Potential predictors of antimanic response to valproate

Diagnosis-related factors	Associated neurological factors
Diagnosis of bipolar disorder (vs. schizoaffective disorder)	Presence of nonparoxysmal EEG abnormalities
Dysphoric (or mixed) mania	Organic affective disorder
Bipolar II disorder	History of closed head trauma
Clinical course variables	Family history
Presence of rapid cycling	Positive family history of mood disorder
Decreasing or stable episode frequency	
Later age at onset of illness	Treatment-related variables
Shorter duration of illness	Patients who are lithium naive
Comorbid psychiatric diagnoses	Higher serum valproate concentrations at days 3–6 of treatment
Comorbid mental retardation	
Comorbid panic attacks	

Note. EEG = electroencephalogram.

Table 6–2. Potential predictors of antidepressant response to valproate

Diagnosis-related factors	Clinical course variables
Diagnosis of bipolar disorder (vs. schizoaffective disorder)	Presence of rapid cycling
Dysphoric (or mixed) mania	Increasing severity of mania
Bipolar II disorder	

schizoaffective disorder, bipolar type. This was first reported by Emrich and colleagues (1985) in a series of patients treated with sodium valproate, carbamazepine, and oxcarbazepine. In a subsequent retrospective review of the records of 73 valproate-treated patients with various psychiatric diagnoses, it was found that 24 of 36 (67%) patients with bipolar disorder had a moderate or marked response to valproate compared with nine of 20 (45%) patients with schizoaffective disorder, in whom only moderate improvement was noted (McElroy et al. 1987, 1988a).

Among patients with bipolar disorder, those with dysphoric or mixed mania (mania associated with depressive symptoms) have been reported to respond favorably to valproate. In a randomized, double-blind, 3-week trial comparing valproate and lithium in the treatment of 27 bipolar patients with acute mania, Freeman and colleagues (1992) found that the presence of high depression scores—defined as at least a 50% reduction in scores on the Schedule for Affective Disorders and Schizophrenia Change Version (SADS-C)—correlated positively with a favorable antimanic response to valproate with an almost fourfold difference in initial SADS-C depression scores and no significant difference in SADS-C mania scores (Clothier et al. 1992; Freeman et al. 1992). Specifically, 9 of 14 (64%) patients with a mean pretreatment SADS-C depression score of 25.6 had a favorable response to valproate (mean posttreatment depression score of 9.0), whereas the remaining 5 patients (36%) who did not respond to valproate had a mean pretreatment SADS-C depression score of 7.0 (mean posttreatment depression score of 9.4). Looking at these results in terms of response rate in mixed versus pure patients, all 4 of the patients diagnosed with mixed mania had a favorable response to valproate, whereas only 5 of 10 pure manic patients responded to valproate. Although this latter group was technically pure, a moderate degree of dysphoria was present based on the mean SADS-C depression scores. Also, it should be noted that 12 of 13 (92%) patients randomized to lithium also had a favorable antimanic response (including six patients who failed at least one previous lithium trial), and that the pretreatment mean SADS-C depression score was 23.6 for this group (posttreatment mean 5.7), which is comparable to the group of patients who responded to valproate. Therefore, although depression severity correlated with antimanic response to valproate, lithium also appeared to be effective in treating patients with dysphoric mania in this study.

The presence of mixed states was associated with an excellent outcome in a cohort of 101 patients with rapid-cycling bipolar disorder treated with open-label valproate for a mean period of 17.2 months (Calabrese and Delucchi 1990; Calabrese et al. 1992, 1993a, 1993b). Forty-three patients received valproate monotherapy, and the remaining 58 patients received valproate in combination with other psychotropics (the majority received lithium and/or carbamazepine). Eight of 10 (80%) patients with mixed mania in the valproate monotherapy group had a marked acute and prophylactic response (complete cessation of symptoms). Thirteen of 15 (87%) patients in the valproate combination therapy group demonstrated a marked acute response, and 16 of 18 (89%) patients demonstrated a marked prophylactic response. Patients with bipolar II disorder (58% of the cohort) had a better acute and prophylactic antimanic response compared with bipolar type I patients. Although this finding reached statistical significance ($P < .03$), the difference in the degree of response was not stated. Nevertheless, this finding suggests that severity of manic symptoms may also be an important factor for valproate response, especially since it was also found that patients with severe mania had a poor outcome.

Favorable antimanic response to valproate was not, however, associated with levels of depression or dysphoria as measured by individual and composite scores on the Brief Psychiatric Rating Scale in a placebo-controlled study of valproate in 36 bipolar patients with acute mania (McElroy et al. 1992). Because controlled trials directly comparing valproate with other mood stabilizers in adequate numbers of patients with well-defined mixed versus nonmixed mania have not yet been conducted, the issue of valproate's increased effectiveness in mixed versus nonmixed mania and whether it is more effective than other agents remains to be definitely proven.

Clinical Course Variables

Several reports have suggested that rapid cycling (the occurrence of four or more affective episodes per year that occurs in 13%–20% of patients with bipolar disorder) may also respond favorably to valproate (Calabrese and Delucchi 1990; Calabrese et al. 1992, 1993a; Herridge and Pope 1985; Keck, Jr. and McElroy 1988; McElroy and Keck Jr 1993b; McElroy et al. 1988b, 1988c). McElroy and colleagues reviewed the records of 38 patients with bipolar disorder treated with valproate at McLean Hospital and identified 6 with rapid cycling (McElroy et al. 1988b). All 6 patients were previously treatment refractory and had received numerous medications including lithium, carbamazepine, and antipsychotics. Marked to moderate improvement was noted in all 6 patients after the addition of valproate to their ongoing medication regimens. Manic episodes decreased in both frequency and severity, with 3 of the 6 patients maintaining a euthymic state for more than a year. Although this was a retrospective review of open-label treatment and concurrent medications were used, the robust response observed in these patients is noteworthy. The cohort of 101 bipolar patients treated with valproate by Calabrese and colleagues have also demonstrated a marked antimanic response. Sixty-four to 74% of patients in short-term treatment and 77%–80% of patients in prophylactic treatment had a marked response to valproate, with 43% of patients receiving valproate monotherapy. Factors potentially limiting the significance of this study include its open design, the use of polypharmacy in many patients, and the reliability on patient reports for outcome measures. Nevertheless, these findings are noteworthy in that the majority of patients were previously unresponsive to conventional treatment with lithium and/or carbamazepine; however, in the controlled study by Pope and colleagues (1991), rapid cycling was not associated with a favorable response to valproate. In the absence of controlled trials directly comparing valproate and other mood stabilizers in adequate numbers of patients with well-defined rapid versus non–rapid-cycling bipolar disorder, it remains unclear whether valproate is more effective in patients who experience rapid cycling than in patients who do not, and whether the drug is more effective than lithium in rapid-cycling bipolar disorder. In the cohort of long-term, prospectively followed patients of Calabrese and colleagues (1993b), decreasing or stable episode frequency was associated with a good antimanic response to valproate. Although this feature may indeed be a legitimate predictor of valproate response, it is likely that patients who are clinically stable and possibly improving would also respond well to lithium or carbamazepine.

Two studies have reported that later ages at onset of illness correlated with a therapeutic response to valproate (Calabrese et al. 1991; McElroy et al. 1991). In a controlled comparison by McElroy and colleagues (1991) of 17 patients with acute mania who were treated with valproate under placebo-controlled, double-blind conditions, the mean age at onset of illness was significantly higher in the 12 patients who responded to valproate (29 years) compared with the 5 patients who did not respond (21 years); however, this finding lost statistical significance when patients who did not respond were compared with a subgroup of 9 who responded markedly, with the mean ages at onset of illness becoming much more similar at 21 and 23 years, respectively. In this same study, shorter duration of illness also correlated with thera-peutic response, but again lost significance when patients who did not respond were compared with patients who responded markedly. It is therefore unclear whether these factors are reliable predictors of response.

Comorbid Psychiatric Diagnoses

Preliminary evidence suggests that there may be an association between valproate response and two comorbid psychiatric diag-noses. In a case series of five patients, valproate was found to be effective in patients with mild to moderate mental retardation and typical ($n = 1$) or atypical ($n = 4$) bipolar disorder (Sovner 1989). Although four of the five patients demonstrated marked improve-ment, this was a diagnostically heterogeneous group, and in-cluded two patients who were autistic (one of whom had also previously sustained a closed head injury), one with Fragile X syndrome, and one with a previous history of major motor sei-zures. Additionally, measures of treatment response were vague, and three of the five patients were receiving antipsychotic drugs concurrently. It is therefore difficult to isolate any individual char-acteristic as a putative predictor of response to valproate. Never-theless, this series does illustrate the potential value of valproate in some very diverse and often treatment-refractory patients.

Bipolar disorder associated with panic attacks may also pref-erentially respond to valproate. In the naturalistic study by Calabrese and Delucchi (1990), panic attacks subsided in 21 of 22 patients (96%) with rapid-cycling bipolar disorder and comor-bid panic disorder who were treated with open-label valproate. Within this group, the number of patients with improvement in affective symptomatology was not stated. Although this point needs clarification, these data, along with studies showing that valproate has antipanic effects in patients with panic disorder, suggest that patients with bipolar disorder and comorbid panic attacks may respond well to valproate, experiencing relief of both affective and panic symptoms (Keck, Jr. et al. 1993a).

Associated Neurological Factors

There are some reports that indicate bipolar patients with associ-ated neurological conditions may respond well to valproate.

McElroy et al. have reported that nonparoxysmal abnormalities on electroencephalogram (EEG) are associated with a therapeutic response to valproate (McElroy et al. 1988a, 1988c, 1992). In reviewing the records of 27 patients who demonstrated a moderate or marked response to valproate, 15 (56%) were found to have nonparoxysmal EEG abnormalities, including 7 patients with localized slowing, 4 with generalized slowing, 3 with brief bursts of higher voltage sharp- and slow-wave activity, and 1 with intermittent background slowing. Conversely, only 5 of 22 (23%) patients who had a minimal or no response to valproate had similar EEG abnormalities; however, there was no association with abnormalities on head computed tomography scans or neurological signs on physical examination. This is noteworthy because closed head trauma has also been associated with a positive response to valproate. In one case series, two patients who developed bipolar disorder after head trauma responded very well to the addition of valproate to their previously mildly effective medication regimens (Pope et al. 1988). In addition, retrospective reviews of patients treated with valproate (added to lithium and neuroleptic regimens) revealed that 7 of 8 (88%) patients with a history of head trauma responded to valproate compared with 22 of 48 (46%) patients without a history of head injury (McElroy et al. 1988c; Pope et al. 1988). Lastly, some patients with organic mood disorder (according to DSM-III-R criteria) have been reported to respond preferentially to valproate. A case series by Kahn and colleagues (1988) involving 3 patients, 2 with a diagnosis of multiple sclerosis and 1 with systemic lupus erythematosus showed, that all 3 patients responded dramatically to valproate therapy after previous treatments had failed.

Family History

Calabrese and colleagues, in their large prospectively followed cohort, also reported that a positive family history of mood disorders predicts a therapeutic response to valproate (Calabrese et al. 1993b). Unfortunately, more specific details such as degree of relatives affected and specific diagnoses were not mentioned. Although this potential predictor of response needs to be validated by further studies, it may provide some valuable insight into the treatment of psychiatric disorders because it takes familial response due to genetic composition into consideration rather than symptom clusters alone.

Treatment-Related Variables

Two treatment-related factors have been found to correlate positively with valproate response. Calabrese and colleagues (1993a) found that rapid-cycling bipolar patients who were lithium naive had a better acute and prophylactic outcome on valproate than patients who had previously received lithium; however, severity of illness and treatment resistance in general may be important confounding factors; it is unclear whether the lithium-naive group was as severely ill. Higher initial serum valproate concentrations may also predict a favorable response to valproate. In analyzing correlations of antimanic response to valproate in patients from the double-blind, placebo-controlled study by Pope and colleagues, the mean serum valproate concentration on days 3–6 of treatment was 53 µg/ml in patients who responded ($n = 12$) compared with 36 µg/ml in patients who did not respond ($n = 5$) (McElroy et al. 1991; Pope et al. 1991). Serum valproate concentrations were not significantly different at the end of the treatment period, suggesting that rapid titration of valproate may have a significant impact on treatment response. This finding was partially replicated in a similar valproate loading study by Keck, Jr. and colleagues, who observed a response (defined as a reduction in MRS scores of more than 50%) in 10 of 19 (53%) patients within 5 days after the initiation of valproate treatment at a dosage of 20 mg/kg/day, achieving a mean serum valproate concentration of 89 ± 19 mg/L on day 2 of treatment (Keck, Jr. et al. 1993b). Therefore, valproate loading or rapid titration of valproate in acute mania may prove to be very useful in achieving a rapid therapeutic response in some patients.

Laboratory-Related Variable

A recent report indicates that for 63 manic patients treated with either valproate, lithium, or placebo for a period of 14–21 days, there was a significant negative correlation between baseline plasma GABA and percent improvement in the Manic Syndrome

Score in patients taking valproate ($r = -.47$, $P = .04$) but not in those taking either lithium or placebo (Petty et al. 1995).

Potential Predictors of Antidepressant Response

Although the antimanic efficacy of valproate is well established, the drug's antidepressant properties are less impressive, especially in the treatment of acute depressive episodes. Since the antidepressant response rate is typically around 30%, it becomes even more important to develop predictors of antidepressant response to valproate so that large numbers of unsuccessful trials may be avoided. The antidepressant efficacy of valproate, however, has not been as systematically studied as its antimanic efficacy, which is reflected in the few open studies done to date. Nevertheless, we will summarize the few findings that have been reported (see Table 6–2).

Diagnosis-Related Factors

As with the antimanic response to valproate, patients with bipolar disorder may be more likely to benefit from the antidepressant properties of valproate than those with schizoaffective disorder. In an open trial of valproate in 15 patients who were followed for a minimum of 26 months, the number of depressive episodes declined 7.7% in patients with bipolar I disorder ($n = 5$) and 83.3% in patients with bipolar II disorder ($n = 5$), although there was a 14.3% increase in the number of depressive episodes in patients with schizoaffective disorder ($n = 5$) (Puzynski and Klosiewicz 1984). This improvement in bipolar type II patients is striking compared with the negligible difference in the other two groups, although the sample size is small. Hayes retrospectively identified 35 patients who received valproate alone or in combination with lithium for an average duration of 1 year, all of whom had previously experienced no improvement with lithium and/or carbamazepine therapy (Hayes 1989). Improvement, defined as an increase in Global Assessment Scale scores, occurred in 12 of 12 patients with mixed mania, compared with 11 of 14 patients with schizoaffective disorder, in whom improvement was not as marked. These response rates are probably artificially elevated due to the use of the Global Assessment Scale as the sole outcome measure, which is nonspecific. Additionally, 6 of 12 bipolar patients and 10 of 14 schizoaffective patients received concurrent lithium. Nevertheless, the strikingly high response rate (100%) in patients with mixed bipolar disorder, while certainly inflated, suggests that this may be a particularly responsive group of patients.

Clinical Course Variables

Clinical course variables that correlate with an antidepressant response to valproate may include the presence of rapid cycling and increasing severity of nonpsychotic mania. In open studies, patients with rapid-cycling bipolar disorder have been reported to display antidepressant responses to valproate, especially prophylactically. In reviewing the records of six consecutive patients with treatment-resistant rapid-cycling bipolar disorder treated with valproate, McElroy and colleagues (1988b) found that all six patients showed marked or moderate improvement after the addition of valproate to their previously minimally or noneffective medication regimen. Improvement in depressive symptomatology and reduction in cycle frequency was observed over the 3–25-month follow-up period. Calabrese and colleagues (1993a) found that 72% of patients who had a marked antimanic response to valproate ($n = 72$) also had a marked (47%) or moderate (25%) prophylactic antidepressant response; however, overall response rates for marked antidepressant efficacy ranged from 21% to 42% in short-term treatment and from 38% to 45% in prophylactic treatment. In addition, Calabrese's group found that the presence of increasingly severe nonpsychotic manic episodes predicted a good acute and prophylactic antidepressant response to valproate.

Conclusion

Valproate, a commonly used anticonvulsant, is becoming a cornerstone in the treatment of bipolar disorder and schizoaffective disorder. Numerous uncontrolled and several controlled studies have demonstrated valproate's efficacy in the treatment of mania, and open studies suggest that it may be effective in preventing manic and depressive episodes. Numerous potential predictors of antimanic response have been identified. These include diagnosis-related factors, including dysphoric mania and bipolar type II disorder; clinical course variables, especially rapid cycling; a family history of mood disorders; associated neurological conditions, including nonparoxysmal EEG abnormalities, organic affective disorders, and a history of closed head trauma; comorbid panic disorder and mental retardation; and treatment-related variables, including high initial serum valproate levels and nonexposure to lithium. Potential predictors of antidepressant response to valproate are more tenuous; however, patients with bipolar depression may respond better than those with schizoaffective depression, and within the bipolar group, patients with dysphoric mania, bipolar type II disorder, and rapid cycling may be the most likely to respond. All of these predictors need to be confirmed by controlled studies. Nevertheless, it is noteworthy that the patient subtypes that respond well to both the antimanic and antidepressant properties of valproate are patients with dysphoric mania, bipolar type II disorder, and rapid cycling. As research continues, further guidelines will become available so that valproate may be used more selectively as responsive populations become better characterized.

References

Brennan MJW, Sandyk R, Borsook D: Use of sodium valproate in the management of affective disorders: basic and clinical aspects, in Anticonvulsants in Affective Disorders. Edited by Emrich HM, Okuma T, Muller AA. Amsterdam, Excerpta Medica, 1984, pp 56–65

Calabrese JR, Delucchi SA: Spectrum of efficacy of valproate in 55 patients with rapid-cycling bipolar disorder. Am J Psychiatry 147:431–434, 1990

Calabrese JR, Markovitz P, Wagner S: Predictors of valproate response in rapid-cycling bipolar disorder. Biol Psychiatry 29:166A–167A, 1991

Calabrese JR, Markovitz PJ, Kimmel SE, et al: Spectrum of efficacy of valproate in 78 rapid-cycling bipolar patients. J Clin Psychopharmacol 12(suppl 1):53S–56S, 1992

Calabrese JR, Woyshville MJ, Kimmel SE, et al: Predictors of valproate response in bipolar rapid cycling. J Clin Psychopharmacol 13:280–283, 1993a

Calabrese JR, Rapport DJ, Kimmel SE, et al: Rapid cycling bipolar disorder and its treatment with valproate. Can J Psychiatry 38(suppl 2):S57–S61, 1993b

Clothier JL, Swann AC, Freeman T: Dysphoric mania. J Clin Psychopharmacol 12:13S–16S, 1992

Emrich HM, Dose M, von Zerrson D: The use of sodium valproate, carbamazepine, and oxcarbazepine in patients with affective disorders. J Affect Disord 8:243–250, 1985

Freeman TW, Clothier JL, Pazzaglia P, et al: A double-blind comparison of valproate and lithium in the treatment of acute mania. Am J Psychiatry 149:108–111, 1992

Hayes SG: Long-term use of valproate in primary psychiatric disorders. J Clin Psychiatry 50(suppl 3):35S–39S, 1989

Herridge PL, Pope HG Jr: Treatment of bulimia and rapid cycling bipolar disorder with sodium valproate: a case report. J Clin Psychopharmacol 5:229–230, 1985

Kahn D, Stevenson E, Douglas CJ: Effect of sodium valproate in three patients with organic brain syndromes. Am J Psychiatry 145:1010–1011, 1988

Keck PE Jr, McElroy SE: Anticonvulsants in the treatment of rapid cycling bipolar disorder, in Use of Anticonvulsants in Psychiatry: Recent Advances. Edited by McElroy SL, Pope HG. Clifton, NJ, Oxford Health Care, 1988

Keck PE Jr, Taylor VE, Tugrul KC, et al: Valproate treatment of panic disorder and lactate-induced panic attacks. Biol Psychiatry 33:542–546, 1993a

Keck PE Jr, McElroy SL, Tugrul KC, et al: Valproate oral loading in the treatment of acute mania. J Clin Psychiatry 54:305–308, 1993b

Lambert P-A: Acute and prophylactic therapies of patients with affective disorders using valpromide (dipropylacetamide), in Anticonvulsant in Affective Disorders. Edited by Emrich HM, Okuma T, Muller AA. Amsterdam, Excerpta Medica, 1984, pp 33–44

Lambert P-A, Cavaz G, Borselli S, et al: Action neuropsychotrop d'un nouvel antiepileptique: le Depamide. Ann Med Psychol 1:707–710, 1966

McElroy SL, Keck PE Jr: Treatment guidelines for valproate in bipolar and schizoaffective disorders. Can J Psychiatry 38:S62–S66, 1993a

McElroy SL, Keck PE Jr: Rapid cycling in Current Psychiatric Therapy. Edited by Dunner DL, WB Saunders, Philadelphia, PA, 1993b, pp 226–231

McElroy SL, Keck PE Jr, Pope HG: Sodium valproate: its use in primary psychiatric disorders. J Clin Psychopharmacol 7:16–24, 1987

McElroy SL, Pope HG, Keck PE Jr, et al: Treatment of psychiatric disorders with valproate: a series of 73 cases. Psychiatr Psychobiol 3:81–85, 1988a

McElroy SL, Keck PE Jr, Pope HG, et al: Valproate in the treatment of rapid-cycling bipolar disorder. J Clin Psychopharmacol 8:275–279, 1988b

McElroy SL, Keck PE Jr, Pope HG, et al: Valproate in primary psychiatric disorders: literature review and clinical experience in a private psychiatric hospital in Use of Anticonvulsants, in Psychiatry: Recent Advances. Edited by McElroy SL, Pope HG. Clifton, NJ, Oxford Health Care, 1988c, pp 25–41

McElroy SL, Keck PE Jr, Pope HG, et al: Correlates of antimanic response to valproate. Psychopharmacol Bull 27:127–133, 1991

McElroy SL, Keck PE Jr, Pope HG, et al: Valproate in the treatment of bipolar disorder: literature review and clinical guidelines. J Clin Psychopharmacol 12:42S–52S, 1992

Penry HK, Dean JC: The scope and use of valproate with epilepsy. J Clin Psychiatry 40(suppl):17–22, 1989

Petty F, Rush AJ, Davis JM, et al: Plasma GABA predicts a response to divalproex sodium in mania (abstract). Biol Psychiatry 37:601, 1995

Pope HG, McElroy SL, Satlin A: Head injury, bipolar disorder, and response to valproate. Compr Psychiatry 29:34–38, 1988

Pope HG, McElroy SL, Keck PE Jr, et al: Valproate in the treatment of acute mania: a placebo-controlled study. Arch Gen Psychiatry 48:62–68, 1991

Puzynski S, Klosiewicz L: Valproic acid amide as a prophylactic agent in affective and schizoaffective disorders. Psychopharmacol Bull 20:151–159, 1984

Sovner R: The use of valproate in the treatment of mentally retarded persons with typical and atypical bipolar disorders. J Clin Psychiatry 50(suppl):40S–43S, 1989

CHAPTER 7

Neuroleptics and Clozapine in Mood Disorders and Schizophrenia

Herbert Y. Meltzer, M.D.,
and S. Hossein Fatemi, M.D., Ph.D.

*A*ntipsychotic drugs, essential in the treatment of schizophrenia, also have an important place in the treatment of mania, psychotic depression, and organic mood disorders. These drugs are especially effective in treating positive and disorganization symptoms (i.e., incoherence, loose associations, inappropriate affect, and poverty of thought content) that may be present in both schizophrenia and mood disorders. To a lesser degree, they are effective in treating negative symptoms in schizophrenia (Meltzer et al. 1986; Opler et al. 1994). Depressive symptoms and negative symptoms may be present in both types of disorders and difficult to distinguish from each other. Nevertheless, neuroleptic drugs, which clearly have antidepressant and antipsychotic effects in psychotic depression, may be unable to prevent the emergence of postpsychotic depression in some patients with

The research reported was supported in part by a grant from the Mental Health Division of the United States Public Health Services (USPHS) (MH41684), a grant from the GCRC (MORR00080), and the National Alliance for Research on Schizophrenia and Depression (NARSAD), as well as grants from the Elisabeth Severance Prentiss, John Pascal Sawyer, and the Stanley Foundations. H.Y.M is the recipient of a USPHS Research Career Scientist Award (MH47808). The secretarial assisstance of Ms. Lee Mason is greatly appreciated.

schizophrenia. This does not rule out the possibility that neuro-leptic drugs also prevent the emergence of depression in other schizophrenic patients recovering from a psychotic exacerbation. The response to antipsychotic drugs in both schizophrenia and mood disorders is quite heterogenous with regard to psycho-pathology as well as other outcome measures. In this chapter we discuss clozapine and atypical antipsychotic drugs that may have superior efficacy for mood disorders compared with typical neuroleptic drugs. Despite their evident advantages, the side ef-fects of neuroleptic drugs (especially extrapyramidal symptoms and tardive dyskinesia), their slow onset of action in some pa-tients, and the agranulocytosis caused by clozapine, make it desirable to identify predictors of response to neuroleptics or clozapine that might enable clinicians to select therapy with these agents and to provide potential risk/benefit assessments to pa-tients. The purpose of this review is to consider selected aspects of the use of typical and atypical antipsychotic drugs and predic-tion of response to both classes of drugs in mood disorders and schizophrenia.

Typical and Atypical Antipsychotic Drugs

It is now customary to divide antipsychotic drugs into two classes: typical and atypical (Meltzer 1992b). Typical antipsychotics in-clude drugs such as haloperidol, fluphenazine, thiothixene, molindone, etc.; these are generally referred to as neuroleptics because of their ability to cause a type of motor impairment known as catalepsy in rodents. The human equivalent of catalepsy, tar-dive dyskinesia symptoms, develops in most, but not all patients, at clinically effective doses. Atypical antipsychotics include drugs that produce markedly fewer tardive dyskinesia symptoms in hu-mans at clinically effective doses. The prototype of an atypical antipsychotic drug is clozapine. Some of the newer antipsychotic drugs such as risperidone and remoxipride (now withdrawn from further development because of its potential to cause aplastic ane-mia) are also atypical. There is debate as to whether thioridazine is atypical since it produces fewer tardive dyskinesia symptoms than other neuroleptics despite sharing many other features with typical neuroleptic drugs. According to a strict definition that focuses on extrapyramidal symptoms, thioridazine should be considered an atypical antipsychotic drug (Meltzer 1994). The typical neuroleptic drugs share a common mechanism of action, the D_2 dopamine receptor blockade. This property is widely regarded as the basis for antipsychotic action as well as for its ability to cause symptoms of tardive dyskinesia. The mechanism of action of atypical antipsychotic drugs is much more complex (Meltzer et al. 1994). Even groups of atypical antipsychotic drugs that share common relevant features, such as weak dopamine D_2 receptor blockade and potent 5-hydroxytryptamine-2A ($5\text{-}HT_{2A}$) receptor blockade (Meltzer et al. 1989), are likely to differ in other important ways, including $5\text{-}HT_6$ and $5\text{-}HT_7$ receptor affinities and M_1 cholinergic receptor affinities (Meltzer et al. 1994; Roth et al. 1994). For this reason, atypical antipsychotic drugs are more apt to be unique with regard to outcome and the most likely predictors of response.

Outcome in Affective Disorders and Schizophrenia

Long-term outcome in affective disorders varies greatly. Approximately 30% of manic-depressive patients have a poor outcome marked by persistent symptomatology, major decrements in social and work function, and frequent relapse and rehospitalization (Goodwin and Jamison 1990; Harrow et al. 1990). There is better overall outcome with major depression but treatment resistance is still frequently encountered (Angst 1988). Major factors predicting poor outcome include premorbid personality disorder, number of episodes, polarity of the disorder (mania worse than depression), earlier age at onset, and male gender (Deister and Marneros 1993).

The diversity in the outcome of schizophrenia, despite treatment with typical or atypical antipsychotics and concomitant psychosocial rehabilitation, is well documented (Ciompi 1980; Harding et al. 1992; Meltzer 1992a, 1992b; McGlashan 1988). The need for a multidimensional perspective on the outcome of schizophrenia has been emphasized (Meltzer 1992a). Outcome studies must look beyond the short-term influence of antipsychotic drugs on psychopathology, and consider, among other measures, cognitive function, social and work function, extrapyramidal function including tardive movement disorders, compliance, suicide rate, rehospitalization, family burden, and cost to society. Each of these outcome measures may, to a degree, be independent of each other, but significant interrelationships also seem likely (Meltzer 1993).

Prediction of response to treatment has generally focused on short-term outcome (weeks to months), whereas long-term outcome is generally referred to as prognosis. The value of predictors of short-term response and prognosis are readily apparent in the face of the great variability in response to treatment, but the multiplicity of relevant response measures and their partial independence make prediction of short-term response and long-term prognosis a complicated matter. Much of the outcome literature for schizophrenia refers to prediction of short-term response (Awad 1989). In this chapter, we consider some of these issues from a clinical perspective.

Typical Neuroleptics in the Treatment of Mania

Several variables must be considered before the institution of antimanic pharmacologic treatment, including severity of illness, presence or absence of other medical disorders, stages and subtypes of mania, and history of drug responsivity (Gerner 1993). A large proportion of manic patients respond well to lithium, carbamazepine, or valproic acid; however, atypical manic states such as dysphoric mania (Clothier et al. 1992), rapid-cycling mania (Dunner 1992), schizoaffective disorder, manic phase (Zelman et al. 1985), mixed mania (Himmelhoch and Garfinkel 1986), organic mania (Nolen 1983), and unipolar mania are less responsive to lithium and more amenable to treatment with valproic acid or carbamazepine (Black et al. 1989; Calabrese et al. 1992; Clothier et al. 1992; Dever and Schweizer 1988; Moller et al. 1989; Post et al. 1987).

In treating mania, the use of other therapies, including neuroleptics, is necessitated by refractoriness to lithium in 20%–40% of manic patients (Chou et al. 1993; Post 1990; Prien and Gelenberg 1989). Multiple factors contribute to lithium refractoriness; these include rapid cycling, severity of symptoms, presence of psychotic features, mixed mania (mania plus depression), secondary mania, organic disorders, negative family history of mood disorders, concomitant substance abuse and dependence, and discontinuation of a previously successful regimen of lithium prophylaxis (Dunner et al. 1976; Post et al. 1987, 1992). Neuroleptics have been used successfully in the treatment of manic patients with clinical features associated with lithium nonresponse, in the rapid behavioral control of agitated patients, in the treatment of elevated mood, and in the treatment of hyperactivity and psychotic symptoms (Chou 1991; Chou et al. 1993). Electroconvulsive treatment (ECT) is also useful in the treatment of mania. Schnur et al. (1992) recently found that high ratings of anger-suspiciousness in medication-nonresponsive manic patients predicted a poor response to ECT.

There is controversy regarding the biological basis of the antimanic effect of neuroleptics as well as the role of increased dopaminergic activity in mania (Gerner 1993; Gerner et al. 1976; Jimerson 1987; Nolen 1983). Silverstone and Cookson (1983) showed that the time course for clinical improvement in manic patients after treatment with either haloperidol or pimozide correlated with an increase in plasma prolactin levels, which is consistent with the antidopaminergic effect of the neuroleptic drugs (Post et al. 1980).

The disadvantages of neuroleptics in treatment of mania include potential for tardive dyskinesia, tardive dyskinesia symptoms, neuroleptic malignant syndrome, possible neurotoxicity secondary to neuroleptic-lithium interaction, inappropriateness in mania prophylaxis, and a subjective feeling of mental dullness that occurs in some patients (Chou 1991; Chou et al. 1993; Gerner 1993).

The Choice of Neuroleptics in Treatment of Mania

Johnson and colleagues (1968, 1971), in a comparison of chlorpromazine and lithium, found lithium to be more effective in the treatment of manic patients; however, other studies (Braden et al. 1982; Prien et al. 1972) have shown chlorpromazine to be more effective than lithium, especially in highly active manic patients.

Overall, more studies report better response to lithium than chlorpromazine (Chou 1991). Additional comparative studies show an equally fast onset of action among chlorpromazine, haloperidol, pimozide, and thioridazine when compared with lithium (Cookson et al. 1981; Post et al. 1980; Prien et al. 1972; Shopsin et al. 1975). These antipsychotics differ in side effects. Thus, Cookson and colleagues (1981) showed that pimozide was less sedating when compared with chlorpromazine. The addition of lithium to neuroleptics does not improve the short-term outcome and does not diminish the need for neuroleptic treatment (Braden et al. 1982; Garfinkel et al. 1980; Johnstone et al. 1988). Moreover, haloperidol alone, or in combination with lithium, has been reported to be superior to lithium alone (Garfinkel et al. 1980).

Neuroleptic Dose-Response in Treatment of Mania

Dosages of neuroleptics in the treatment of mania have varied widely; for example, mean haloperidol doses have ranged from 16.4 mg/day (Juhl et al. 1977), to 24 mg/day (Chou 1991), to 48 mg/day (Krishna et al. 1978), and up to 90 mg/day (Shopsin et al. 1975). According to Janicak and colleagues (1988), these doses are probably excessive and have the potential to produce tardive dyskinesia if continued. These authors also reported that moderately low doses of neuroleptics are sufficient to control most acute manic episodes during the lag period before lithium takes full effect (Cohen et al. 1980; Janicak et al. 1988). Janicak's group hypothesized that the dose-response curve for maintenance treatment of mania was similar to that for schizophrenia; if so, doses of 5–10 mg/day of haloperidol should be adequate. Additional reports (Chou et al. 1993; Rifkin et al. 1990) have confirmed the previous work done by Janicak and colleagues (1988), showing that low-dose neuroleptics (i.e., haloperidol 10 mg/day) can be effective in the treatment of psychosis in acute mania and in the maintenance treatment of manic patients (Chou et al. 1993).

The use of neuroleptics in the long-term treatment of mania has been recently reviewed by Sernyak and Woods (1993). These authors note that their use is surprisingly widespread, and provide estimates of 40%–42% for maintenance treatment and 90%–

100% for any exposure; however, there is considerable variability. One community sample in Los Angeles reported almost no use of neuroleptics (Escobar et al. 1987). Sernyak and Woods (1993) found little evidence for an advantage to chronic use of neuroleptics in mania and discouraged it because of the risk of tardive dyskinesia, noncompliance, and neuroleptic malignant syndrome. A retrospective study comparing relapse rates in manic patients receiving depot neuroleptic drugs (i.e., given by intramuscular depot injection for 2–4 weeks at a time) suggested that this approach may be useful as a supplement to lithium or carbamazepine, or as a sole treatment (White et al. 1993).

Clinical practice has suggested that patients who relapse frequently despite being on mood stabilizers may be the best candidates for neuroleptics; however, the ever-present danger of tardive dyskinesia must be kept in mind. This suggests the wider use of atypical antipsychotic drugs such as clozapine or perhaps risperidone instead of typical neuroleptic drugs. We will discuss this topic in more detail later on in the chapter.

Predictors of Response to Neuroleptics in Bipolar Mood Disorders

A survey of the literature concerning predictors of response to neuroleptics in bipolar patients reveals a paucity of information. In several papers published by Taylor and Abrams (1973, 1975, 1977, 1981), a variety of factors were investigated that dealt with the responsiveness of patients with mania to somatic therapies and ECT. In their earliest work, these authors showed that the presence of catatonia or first-rank symptoms did not predict a poor outcome for manic patients. Furthermore, the number of patients with marked response or full remission after treatment with lithium alone, neuroleptics alone, or a combination of both did not vary considerably. Unfortunately, no dose-response parameters were given (Taylor and Abrams 1973). In a second study, these authors suggested that the presence of euphoric mood, grandiose delusional ideas, cyclothymic premorbid personality, and a family history of affective disease may be useful as predictors of treatment response to the same combination of medications, especially in an acute manic state (Taylor and Abrams 1975).

In their third study, these authors suggested that catatonic signs are nonspecific and may be highly prevalent among patients with bipolar affective disease (Taylor and Abrams 1977). Finally, Taylor and Abrams (1981) evaluated the response to somatic treatments (placebo, lithium alone, neuroleptic alone, lithium and neuroleptics, or ECT in combination with or without medications) in a sample of 111 manic patients using multiple outcome measures. The variables included age at onset, current age, duration of index hospital stay, duration of index episode, admission severity score, male/female ratio, episodes per patient per year, electroencephalogram (EEG) studies, neuropsychological tests, and family and historical information. They concluded that except for a positive, perhaps unimportant, relationship between abnormal EEG and improvement, there was no evidence for biological differences between patients who did and did not respond to treatment (Taylor and Abrams 1981). Goodwin and Jamison (1990) have criticized this report for the authors' sole reliance on clinicians' recommendations regarding use of various treatment modalities for patients with different clinical profiles and have cautioned against drawing any conclusions concerning prediction of treatment response.

A recent prospective 10-year follow-up study of 131 bipolar patients demonstrated no clear effect of various treatment modalities on the course of bipolar disease (Winokur et al. 1994). The treatment modalities included antipsychotics, antidepressant, and antimanic agents (no information about neuroleptic type, dosage, and time course was given). In a period of 5 years, it was demonstrated that intensity of treatment did not affect the cycle length or the number of episodes. Thus, in spite of treatment provided to most patients, treatment modality was not a predictive variable for the course of bipolar illness. There was, however, an interaction between treatment intensity and the number of hospitalizations, but this may have been due simply to the increase in treatment intensity during each hospitalization. Additionally, these authors found that 1) no difference existed in the number of episodes between men and women, 2) alcoholism showed a great diminution at the end of 10 years, 3) cycle lengths showed no decrease in length over the 10-year period, 4) cycle lengths and the number of episodes in the first 5 years and the last 5 years were similar, 5) family history of mania was associated with more episodes at follow-up, 6) patients with alcoholism predating the onset of their bipolar disorder were less likely to have episodes during the follow-up period than patients in whom bipolar disorder predated the onset of alcoholism, and 7) chronicity (absence of any 8-week period of wellness) from the index episode to the end of the 10-year follow-up was uncommon (4%).

The Role of Neuroleptics in Treatment of Psychotic Depression

Psychotic depression is a major depressive episode accompanied by hallucinations, delusions, or a combination thereof (Akiskal and Puzantian 1979; Black and Nasrallah 1989; Frances et al. 1981). The treatment response rate to tricyclic antidepressants and monoamine oxidase inhibitors ranges from 20% to 30% (Dubovsky and Thomas 1992). Various reports indicate that 19%–48% of patients with psychotic depression respond to treatment with neuroleptics alone (Spiker et al. 1985, 1986; Khan et al. 1987). The addition of antidepressants to neuroleptics increases the response rate to 70%–80% (Dubovksy and Thomas 1992). The presumed mechanisms of action behind combination therapy is complex and may involve various neurotransmitters. A report by Mikuni and Meltzer (1984) showed augmented reduction of $5-HT_2$ binding sites in rat cortex by the combination of imipramine and chlorpromazine. The doses of neuroleptics used in the treatment of psychotic depression are markedly variable. These may be moderate (10–20 mg/day of haloperidol equivalent) (Dubovsky and Thomas 1992; Khan et al. 1987; Minter and Mandel 1979) or high (40 mg/day of haloperidol equivalent or more) (Aronson et al. 1988; Nelson et al. 1986; Spiker et al. 1985, 1986). It is likely that high-dose neuroleptic treatment will cause more side effects and may actually result in poorer treatment response in mania. As with schizophrenia, lower doses should be tried for periods of 4–8 weeks before being increased.

Predictors of Response to Neuroleptics

The factors that have been shown in more than one study to predict short-term response to neuroleptic drugs as well as better long-term outcome in schizophrenia have some overlap and are listed in Table 7–1. Some of these have been reviewed by Awad (1989) and Lieberman and Sobel (1993).

The clinical predictors in Table 7–1 (i.e., older age at onset, few negative symptoms) may be useful in a general sense to alert clinicians to expect good results from neuroleptic treatment in both first-episode patients with schizophrenia as well as patients experiencing recurrent episodes in chronic schizophrenia. For first-episode patients, the main predictors of good outcome are good premorbid adjustment, abrupt onset, presence of mainly positive and few negative symptoms, and possibly a shorter duration of illness before treatment initiation (Awad 1989; Wyatt 1991). For chronic schizophrenic patients, the best predictors of response are usually previous response to neuroleptic drugs and

Table 7–1. Factors associated with better short- and long-term response to typical neuroleptic drugs

- History of good response to neuroleptics
- Female gender
- Negative family history of schizophrenia
- Absence of childhood asociality
- High level of functioning before onset
- Later age at onset
- Abrupt onset
- Rapid initiation of treatment after onset
- Precipitating events
- Mainly positive symptoms
- Affective symptoms
- Few negative symptoms
- Paranoid subtype
- Compliance with drug treatment
- Fewer previous hospitalizations
- Plasma levels of neuroleptics
- Absence of cortical atrophy or ventricular enlargement
- Increased plasma homovanillic acid (HVA)
- Enhanced growth hormone response to apomorphine

history of compliance with drug treatment; however, there are many exceptions to these generalizations.

Many patients show mixtures of good and poor predictors of outcome. Therefore, it is of interest to attempt a multivariate approach to the prediction of response. While this may not be practical for clinical purposes, it can shed light on possible subtypes of schizophrenia for research purposes. An example of this, albeit unsuccessful, was the type I/II model of Crow (1980), which linked negative symptoms, absence of positive symptoms, and large ventricles to poor response, and linked absence of ventricular enlargement to good response to typical neuroleptics. As has been discussed elsewhere, these elements may be independent of each other (Meltzer 1985). In a recent Hungarian study, Bartkó and colleagues (1990) examined 22 putative sociodemographic, psychosocial, clinical, neurocognitive, and biochemical predictors of response in 98 schizophrenic patients hospitalized for relapse. The mean age was 37.5 years (range, 19–58), the mean duration of illness was 10.5 years (range, 4–17), the mean number of hospitalizations was 6.2 (range, 2–11), and the mean length of education was 11.3 years (range, 6–17). After admission, patients were treated with neuroleptics, mainly haloperidol, with a mean dose of 615 ± 320 mg/day of chlorpromazine equivalents. The minimum dose was the equivalent of 400 mg/day of chlorpromazine with no high-dosage treatment in any case. Treatment outcome at 28 days was assessed by the consensus of two psychiatrists using a 4-point scale (1 = very good response, 4 = no/poor response). Each of the 22 items was correlated with outcome, then a stepwise multiple regression analysis was used.

After 28 days, 35 patients (35.7%) showed a very good response, 29 (29.6%) a good response, 26 (26.5%) a fair response, and 8 (9.2%) a poor response. Of the 22 predictors, the following 10 were significantly correlated with a good outcome (in order of most significant correlation): 1) less disturbance of premorbid adjustment, 2) greater intensity of positive symptoms, 3) less impairment of working ability, 4) short duration of previous hospitalization, 5) young age at first hospitalization, 6) living with family or in a social environment, 7) absence of family history of schizophrenia, 8) quality of social contacts, 9) low serum dopamine β-hydroxylase activity, and 10) severity of tardive dyskinesia. The five items that predicted 20% of outcome variance with

cumulative percent of variance explained were: 1) less disturbance of premorbid adjustment (11%), 2) greater intensity of positive symptoms at admission (18%), 3) absence of family history of
schizophrenia (23%), 4) less impairment of working ability (27%),
and 5) low serum dopamine β-hydroxylase activity (29%). The
following factors did not predict outcome: age, gender, length of
education, duration of illness, number of previous hospitalizations, stressful life events, time of onset of psychopathology
before admission, handedness, neurological soft signs, abnormal
voluntary movements, cognitive impairment, and spontaneous
blink rate. These results are only for response to 4 weeks of
neuroleptic treatment. The results, although quite interesting, are
illustrative of the problems with the prediction literature, because
those factors generally thought to predict response (sex, duration
of illness, and time of onset of psychopathological features) did
not predict outcome in this study.

In a recent study of first-break patients, Lieberman and colleagues (1992a) found that duration of psychotic symptoms was
the only variable studied that had an independent significant effect on time to remission. They suggested that these results were
consistent with a group of studies (see Wyatt 1991) that had found
duration of illness before treatment correlated with poor outcome. Baseline severity of positive or negative symptoms did not
predict outcome, but the deficit state identified by Carpenter and
colleagues (1988) predicted a poor outcome. Male sex, early age
at onset, poor premorbid level of function, and longer duration
of illness were also predictive of poor response. The possibility
that delay in initiation of treatment may have an adverse effect
on outcome for the current episode as well as throughout the
course of illness would, if true, have a powerful influence on the
importance of and the ability to identify other predictors that
might be independent of this effect. Future studies must establish
this point for clinical purposes as well as to facilitate valid research
outcome.

Studies of predictors of long-term response have been extensively reviewed by McGlashan (1988). More recent studies of
prognostic factors, summarized by Lieberman and Sobel (1993),
continue to identify predictors of poor outcome such as young
age at onset (less than 19 years old) (Gmur 1991; Tsoi and Wong
1991); poor premorbid function (Carpenter and Strauss 1991; Leff

et al. 1992; Tien and Eaton 1992); duration of illness longer than 6 months prior to treatment (Leff et al. 1992; Tsoi and Wong 1991); insidious onset (Schmid et al. 1991); poor short-term response to typical neuroleptics (Carpenter and Strauss 1991; Gmur 1991; Marengo et al. 1991), including persistence of negative symptoms (Fenton and McGlashan 1991a) or negative and positive symptoms (Breier et al. 1991); male sex (Leff et al. 1992); absence of affective symptoms (Grossman et al. 1991); undifferentiated, catatonic, or hebephrenic subtype (Fenton and McGlashan 1991b); and ventricular enlargement (DeLisi et al. 1992; Lieberman et al. 1992b; Vita et al. 1991).

Biological Predictors of Response to Neuroleptic Drugs in Schizophrenia

Numerous studies have sought to identify biological predictors of response to neuroleptic drugs. In part, these are based on etiological hypotheses of schizophrenia, such as excesses of dopaminergic or noradrenergic activity, hypoglutamatergic activity, increased serotonergic activity, and structural brain abnormalities. For example, there are a number of reports that state that increased baseline plasma homovanillic acid (HVA) may predict treatment response to standard neuroleptic drugs (Bowers et al. 1984; Chang et al. 1980; Mazure et al. 1991) or that the decrease in plasma HVA during neuroleptic treatment correlates with clinical response (Mazure et al. 1991; Pickar et al. 1986).

Friedman and colleagues (1992) conducted a meta-analysis of 33 studies relating the clinical response to typical neuroleptic drugs to the ventricular brain ratio. No overall relationship was found. There is considerable evidence that cortical sulcal prominence does not predict response to typical neuroleptic drugs (Boronow et al. 1985; Naber et al. 1985; Nasrallah et al. 1983; Nimgaonkar et al. 1988; The Scottish Schizophrenia Research Group et al. 1989; Smith et al. 1987; Vita et al. 1988), although one study did report such a relationship (Smith et al. 1983).

Neuroleptic plasma levels have been intensively studied as a predictor of response to neuroleptic drugs (see Van Putten et al. 1991 for review). Haloperidol and fluphenazine have been the most frequently studied. The results are conflicting. There is some evidence for a therapeutic window with haloperidol, but many patients with high plasma levels do not appear to be adversely affected. In general, measurement of plasma levels of typical neuroleptic drugs are not warranted in clinical practice.

Clozapine

Clozapine is an atypical antipsychotic drug that is indicated for use in neuroleptic-resistant schizophrenic patients, that is, patients who have failed to show a satisfactory response to typical neuroleptic drugs, or patients who are neuroleptic-intolerant (e.g., have moderate to severe Parkinsonian side effects such as akathisia, rigidity, stiffness, or tardive movement disorders, despite using the lowest doses of a typical neuroleptic like thioridazine, with relatively low potential to cause extrapyramidal symptoms). It is estimated that 15%–30% of schizophrenic patients are neuroleptic resistant according to the strict criteria of moderate to severe psychopathology despite neuroleptic trials of adequate duration with at least three typical neuroleptic drugs of different chemical classes; however, at least 60% of the remaining 70%–85% of patients with schizophrenia have a quality of life that is very compromised in terms of social and work function and sense of well-being (Helgason 1990). Thus, a broader definition of neuroleptic resistance has been advocated (Meltzer 1992b). Some patients with schizophrenia are neuroleptic intolerant from the first episode, whereas others do not become intolerant until later in the course of illness (Kolakowska et al. 1975; Loebel et al. 1992).

The use of clozapine is restricted mainly because it causes granulocytopenia or agranulocytosis in .75%–1.0% of cases (Alvir et al. 1993; Krupp and Barnes 1989). Despite this side effect liability, the advantages of clozapine are sufficient to outweigh the risks in many cases of schizophrenia, especially since the possibility of morbidity and mortality may be minimized by weekly monitoring of the white blood cell count. Prompt discontinuation of clozapine when granulocytopenia or agranulocytosis occurs leads to a reversal of the hematologic complication in almost all cases. The overall mortality is 1:10,000 (.01%) (Alvir et al. 1993); this must be balanced against the risk of death in schizophrenia due to other causes such as suicide (9%–12% lifetime for schizophrenia, and occurring at the rate of .4%–.8%/year) (Meltzer and Okayli 1995). Because clozapine is used primarily in neuroleptic-resistant patients, predictors of response to typical neuroleptic drugs are not likely to be valid predictors of response to clozapine.

The study of Meltzer and colleagues established the efficacy of clozapine in neuroleptic-resistant schizophrenic patients (Kane et al. 1988). This involved nearly 300 neuroleptic-resistant patients who were randomly assigned to receive either clozapine or chlorpromazine for 6 weeks after an open trial of haloperidol failed to alleviate symptoms. Thirty percent of the clozapine-treated patients responded versus 3% of the chlorpromazine-treated patients using predetermined criteria for this categorical distinction. Patients who responded to clozapine had to be only mildly ill in terms of psychopathology or overall function.

Honigfeld and Patin (1989) used multiple regression to find predictors of outcome in the clozapine-treated group, followed by discriminant function analysis to determine whether patients could be categorized into response and nonresponse groups. Demographic, diagnostic, historical, and symptomatic variables were evaluated. Patients who met DSM-III criteria for paranoid subtype (295.3) were found to respond better, but this accounted for only 5.4% of the variance. Among the demographic characteristics, a greater number of previous hospitalizations predicted better response, accounting for 2.9% of the variance. Duration of illness, duration of current episode, age at first hospitalization, length of current hospitalization, and severity of tardive dyskinesia did not predict response. Each of the 18 items in the Brief Psychiatric Rating Scale (BPRS) (Overall and Gorham 1962) was evaluated as a predictor. Low grandiosity was a favorable pretreatment characteristic and accounted for 2.9% of outcome variance. Negative symptoms assessed by the Schedule for Assessment of Negative Symptoms (SANS) did not contribute. The three predictors noted above accounted for 13.3% of outcome variance. Discriminant function using these measures produced unsatisfactory prediction (about 30% false characterization).

The authors have also found that sex and duration of illness predict response to clozapine depending on the time of assessment of response and the outcome measure. Thus, being female and having a shorter duration of illness may sometimes predict a better response to clozapine. It has also been found that having tardive dyskinesia may predict a better response to clozapine (Meltzer, in press). These effects, however, are relatively modest and account for only a small amount of variance.

Pickar and colleagues (1992) reported that later age at onset and greater decrease in Parkinsonian side effects on clozapine, compared with baseline levels on fluphenazine, predicted good response to clozapine. There is also considerable evidence that weight gain is a side effect of clozapine (Cohen et al. 1990; Lamberti et al. 1992). Lamberti and colleagues (1992) reported a trend for the decrease in BPRS scores in 30 patients treated with clozapine for 6 months to be inversely correlated with weight gain (17 lbs on average; Spearman $\rho = -.31, P < .10$).

Plasma levels of clozapine, which are nonlinearly dose dependent, have recently been reported to predict response to clozapine. Three early European studies produced negative results (Ackenheil et al. 1976; Brau et al. 1978; Thorup and Fog 1977), but these studies can be criticized for design flaws and limited sample size. Perry and colleagues (1991) were the first to report that plasma levels of clozapine were positively related to clinical response. In this study, 29 neuroleptic-resistant patients were treated with clozapine at a fixed dose of 400 mg/day. This dose produced a mean clozapine plasma concentration 4 weeks after reaching 400 mg/day of 348 ± 307 ng/ml. N-desmethylclozapine levels were 111 ± 92 ng/ml. Plasma levels 4 weeks after reaching maximum dose were used for analysis. Eleven of the 29 patients responded. Patients who did not respond had higher baseline BPRS scores. The mean clozapine levels of patients who responded were 404 ± 123 ng/ml versus 356 ± 255 ng/ml for patients who did not respond ($P = $ NS). The mean norclozapine levels were 123 ± 70 ng/ml and 112 ± 63 ng/ml, respectively ($P = $ NS); however, using a receiver operating characteristic analysis, it was found that plasma levels of clozapine greater than or equal to 350 ng/ml produced the best differentiation of response (7 of 11, 63.6%) from nonresponse (14 of 18, 77.8%).

The authors' laboratory studied plasma clozapine levels at a random period in 59 clozapine-treated schizophrenic patients (Hasegawa et al. 1993). This included 30 patients who responded and 29 who did not. The mean dose of clozapine in the two groups was 460 ± 184 mg/day and 429 ± 143 mg/day, respectively ($P = $ .54); however, plasma clozapine levels were 440 ± 274 ng/ml and

300 ± 200 ng/ml, respectively ($P = .03$). Plasma norclozapine levels were also significantly lower in the patients who did not respond ($P = .02$). Using discriminant function analysis, a clozapine plasma concentration value of 370 ng/ml was determined to be the optimal cutoff to classify patients who responded and patients who did not. A receiver operating characteristic curve produced the same result with a 67.5% efficiency in classification. Similar results have now been found by two other laboratories (J. Lieberman, personal communication; S. Potkin, personal communication). These results suggest that to optimize the response to clozapine, plasma levels of clozapine of 350 ng/ml or higher should be sought.

Prefrontal Sulcal Prominence as a Predictor of Response to Clozapine

The authors' laboratory (Friedman et al. 1991) reported that increased prefrontal cortical sulcal widening (PFSW) predicted a poor response to clozapine at 6 weeks in 26 neuroleptic-resistant schizophrenic patients. Patients were classified as having no response or a moderate response (15%–40% decrease in BPRS scores from baseline) and as having a good response (a decrease of 40% or more in BPRS scores) based on a cluster analysis of BPRS scores at baseline and 6 weeks after initiation of clozapine. There was a highly significant linear trend relating better response to lower PFSW. The same relationship held for the BPRS subscales of thought disorder, positive symptoms, negative symptoms, and paranoid disturbance. Similar results were obtained with a multiple regression model. Ventricular brain ratio and third ventricle width did not predict response to clozapine. Friedman and colleagues (1992) conducted a meta-analysis of 33 studies relating clinical response to typical neuroleptics to ventricular brain ratio. No overall relationship was found. Recently, Schröder and colleagues (1993) studied brain images of 50 schizophrenic patients using computed tomography. Twenty-one patients who were neuroleptic resistant or neuroleptic intolerant were treated with clozapine, whereas 20 were treated with typical neuroleptics. During a mean 30-day treatment period, there was a significant correlation between decrease in total BPRS score and average width of the three largest cortical sulci ($\rho = -.46$, $P > .005$). The BPRS Thought Disorder subscale was also correlated with this measure. The change in BPRS score was also inversely related to frontal horn ratio, third ventricle width, ventricular ratio, and width of frontal interhemispheric feature. These relationships applied to both treatments. The authors' early results with clozapine were thus replicated.

The robustness of the relationship between PFSW and response to clozapine suggests that this measure may be of some value in clinical practice. In the study by Friedman and colleagues (1991), 14.7% of the variance in total BPRS scores at 6 weeks was explained by PFSW, and another 16% was explained by baseline BPRS scores. Thus, high PFSW could be used to identify change of response to clozapine by 6 weeks. The frontal lobe has also been implicated in response to clozapine by Small and colleagues (1987), who reported that patients who responded to clozapine had higher EEG alpha amplitude in frontal and temporal areas than patients who did not respond.

Neurochemical Predictors of Response to Clozapine

Several biological indices have been suggested to be predictors of response to clozapine. Pickar and colleagues (1992) reported that plasma HVA levels were significantly lower during clozapine treatment in patients who had a good response to clozapine ($n = 8$) versus those patients with less response ($n = 13$) ($P = .07$). They also found that the patients who had a good respond to clozapine had lower cerebrospinal fluid levels of HVA/5-hydroxyindoleacetic acid (HVA/5-HIAA) while receiving typical neuroleptics, during a placebo washout, or on clozapine. They suggested that this finding was consistent with a serotonin-dopamine imbalance as a determinant of clozapine action, as the authors had previously suggested (Meltzer 1989). Szymanski and colleagues (1993) also reported that pretreatment cerebrospinal fluid HVA/5-HIAA ratio, and, to a lesser extent, the cerebrospinal fluid HVA levels, predicted treatment response to clozapine.

Green and colleagues (1993), like Pickar and colleagues (1992), found that pretreatment plasma HVA strongly correlated with the total BPRS score and BPRS positive symptoms. They reported that pretreatment plasma HVA levels at baseline correlated with the clinical response to clozapine at 3 months; however, they failed to adjust the response for baseline levels, so this result may be spurious. Davidson and colleagues (1993) found no effect of clozapine on plasma HVA and no relationship between change in plasma HVA levels and response to clozapine. The authors have also found no relationship between response to clozapine and change in plasma HVA (unpublished results). Such studies require attention to such factors as baseline level of psychopathology and other predictors such as prefrontal atrophy and duration of illness.

There have been several efforts to relate response to clozapine to subtypes of D_4 receptors; these have produced negative results with the exception of some unpublished data from this laboratory in conjunction with James Kennedy, M.D., Ph.D., at the University of Toronto. Specific isoforms of the D_4 gene that are related to better response to clozapine have been found.

Clozapine and Mood Disorders

There is a body of evidence that indicates that clozapine is effective in a variety of mood disorders. Before the risk of agranulocytosis was known, clozapine was used to treat endogenous depression (Nahunek et al. 1975). Patients who responded best in that study were re-sorted to include those with marked anxiety, agitation, and some atypical features. Treatment-resistant depressed patients (i.e., those who fail to respond to tricyclic antidepressants, neuroleptics, or ECT) have been found to respond to clozapine (Dassa et al. 1993; Parsa et al. 1991). There are also a number of studies indicating the efficacy of clozapine in refractory bipolar and schizoaffective disorders (Calabrese et al. 1991, 1994; McElroy et al. 1991; Naber and Hippius 1990; Suppes et al. 1992). The use of clozapine in the treatment of schizoaffective disorders has recently been reviewed (Keck Jr et al. 1994). There are no specific predictors of response within this refractory group of mood disorders. It is clear that clozapine should be used only after standard therapies have been tried or because of the presence of tardive dyskinesia or dystonia. Given the risk of tardive movement disorder in patients with mood disorders, clozapine or other low extrapyramidal symptom–producing antipsychotics should be considered whenever tardive dyskinesia is a concern. There is no evidence yet that risperidone is effective in mania or schizoaffective disorders, but it seems likely that it will be tried for these indications and may prove to be superior to typical neuroleptic drugs with regard to extrapyramidal side effects.

Risperidone

Risperidone is another atypical antipsychotic approved for treatment of schizophrenia by the FDA in 1994 with combined anti-dopamine and antiserotonin activity (Borison et al. 1992). At this time, there have been a series of reports on the application of risperidone successfully to mania (Ghaemi et al. 1995, Goodnick 1995; Singh and Catalan 1994; Tohen et al. 1995), to rapid-cycling disorder (Jacobsen 1995), and to psychotic depression (Hillert et al. 1992). Singh and Catalan looked at four patients with HIV-related mania and reported reductions in the Young Mania Scale (YMS) score of approximately 75% within 7–10 days. Goodnick has found normalization of DSM-III-R mania at doses of 3–6 mg/day within several days and practically total resolution within 1 week. Tohen and coworkers reported in 12 patients given 2–6 mg/day for 6 weeks for psychotic mania, nine (75%) showed at least 75% decrease in the YMS. Ghaemi and colleagues indicated that adjunctive risperidone produced a further 64% rate of improvement for outpatient bipolar disorder. Jacobsen showed that 85% of patients (mostly bipolar) had decreases in agitation, psychosis, sleep disturbance, and rapid cycling. Hillert and coworkers found that 2–10 mg/day for 6 weeks resulted in 70% of patients with psychotic depression showing significant resolution of all symptoms. Where patients presented with mixed mood symptoms, Dwight and coworkers (1994) found a risk of risperidone-treatment associated onset of manic symptoms in three patients. Overall, Keck and coworkers (1995) recently reported that among 49 patients with schizophrenia, 81 with schizoaffective (58 bipolar, 23 depressive type), and 11 with bipolar disorder that moderate to marked treatment response was associated with younger age, diagnoses of bipolar disorder and depressive-type schizoaffective

disorder, shorter duration of illness, and shorter length of hospitalization before receiving risperidone.

Conclusion

In conclusion, the heterogeneity in response to neuroleptic treatment or clozapine makes it desirable to evaluate predictors of response to either form of treatment. Such predictors do not act in
isolation and may be influenced by each other as well as other
treatment modalities. Among the relevant modalities are sex, age
at onset, duration of illness, family history, and biological factors
such as genetics, structural brain changes, and plasma HVA. Nevertheless, there are no absolutely definitive predictors of response.
Clinical trials are essential to establish efficacy in many cases. Previous history of drug response is the best guide in more chronic
cases.

References

Ackenheil VM, Brau H, Burkhart A, et al: Antipsychotic efficacy in relation
   to plasma levels of clozapine. Arzneimittelforschung 26:1156–1158,
   1976

Akiskal HS, Puzantian VR: Psychotic forms of depression and mania. Psychiatr Clin North Am 2:419–439, 1979

Alvir JMJ, Lieberman JA, Safferman AZ, et al: Clozapine-induced agranulocytosis incidence and risk factors in the United States. N Engl J Med
   329:162–167, 1993

Angst J: Clinical course of affective disorders, in Depressive Illness: Predictor of Course and Outcome. Edited by Helgason T, Daly TJ. Berlin,
   Springer-Verlag, 1988

Aronson TA, Shukla S, Hoff A: Continuation therapy after ECT for delusional depression: a naturalistic study of prophylactic treatments and
   relapse. Convulsive Ther 3:251–259, 1988

Awad G: Drug therapy in schizophrenia: variability of outcome and prediction of response. Can J Psychiatry 34:711–720, 1989

Bartkó G, Frecska E, Horvath S, et al: Predicting neuroleptic response from
   a combination of multilevel variables in acute schizophrenic patients.
   Acta Psychiatr Scand 82:408–412, 1990

Black DW, Nasrallah A: Hallucinations and delusions in 1715 patients with
   unipolar and bipolar affective disorders. Psychopathology 22:28–34,
   1989

Black DW, Hulbert J, Nasrallah A: The effect of somatic treatment and comorbidity on immediate outcome in manic patients. Compr Psychiatry 30:74–79, 1989

Borison RL, Diamond BL, Pathiraja A: Clinical overview of risperidone, in Novel Antipsychotic Drugs. Edited by Meltzer HY. New York, Raven, 1992, pp 233–239

Boronow J, Pickar D, Ninan PT, et al: Atrophy limited to the third ventricle in chronic schizophrenic patients. Arch Gen Psychiatry 42:266–271, 1985

Bowers MB Jr, Swigar ME, Jatlow PI, et al: Plasma catecholamine metabolites and early response to haloperidol. J Clin Psychiatry 45:248–251, 1984

Braden W, Fink EB, Qualls CB, et al: Lithium and chlorpromazine in psychotic inpatients. Psychiatry Res 7:69–81, 1982

Brau VH, Burkhart A, Pacho W, et al: Beziehungen zwischen Wirkungen und Plasmaspiegeln von Clozapin. Arzneim-Forsch/Drug Res 28:1300–1301, 1978

Breier A, Schreiber JL, Dyer J, et al: National Institute of Mental Health longitudinal study of chronic schizophrenia. Arch Gen Psychiatry 48:239–246, 1991

Calabrese JR, Meltzer HY, Markovitz PJ: Clozapine prophylaxis in rapid cycling: bipolar disorder. J Clin Psychopharmacol 11:396–397, 1991

Calabrese JR, Markovitz PJ, Kimmel SE, et al: Spectrum of efficacy of valproate in 78 rapid-cycling bipolar patients. J Clin Psychopharmacol 12:535–565, 1992

Calabrese J, Kimmel SE, Woyshville M, et al: Clozapine in treatment-refractory mania. Am J Psychiatry (in press)

Carpenter WT Jr, Strauss JS: The prediction of outcome in schizophrenia, IV: eleven year follow up of the Washington IPSS cohort. J Nerv Ment Dis 179:517–525, 1991

Carpenter WT Jr, Heinrichs DW, Wagman AMI. Deficit and nondeficit forms of schizophrenia: the concept. Am J Psychiatry 145:578–583, 1988

Chang W-H, Chen T-Y, Lin S-K, et al: Plasma catecholamine metabolites in schizophrenics: evidence for the subtype concept. Biol Psychiatry 27:510–518, 1980

Chou JCY: Recent advances in treatment of acute mania. J Clin Psychopharmacol 11:3–21, 1991

Chou JCY, Tuma I, Sweeney EA: Treatment approaches for acute mania. Psychiatr Q 54:331–344, 1993

Ciompi L: The natural history of schizophrenia in the long term. Br J Psychiatry 136:413–420, 1980

Clothier J, Swann A, Freeman T: Dysphoric mania. J Clin Psychopharmacol 12:135–165, 1992

Cohen BM, Lipinski JF, Pope HG: Neuroleptic blood levels and therapeutic effects. Psychopharmacology 70:191–193, 1980

Cohen LJ, Test MA, Brown RL: Suicide and schizophrenia: data from a prospective community treatment study. Am J Psychiatry 147:602–607, 1990

Cookson J, Silverstone T, Wells B: Double-blind comparative clinical trial of pimozide and chlorpromazine in mania. Acta Psychiatr Scand 64:381–397, 1981

Crow TJ: Molecular pathology of schizophrenia: more than one disease process? BMJ 280:66–68, 1980

Dassa D, Kaladjian A, Azorin JM, et al: Clozapine in the treatment of psychotic refractory depression. Br J Psychiatry 163:822–824,1993

Davidson M, Kahn RS, Stern RG, et al: Treatment with clozapine and its effect on plasma homovanillic acid and norepinephrine concentrations in schizophrenia. Psychiatry Res 46:151–164, 1993

Deister A, Marneros A: Predicting the long-term outcome of affective disorders. Acta Psychiatr Scand 88:174–177, 1993

DeLisi LE, Strizke P, Riordan H, et al: The timing of brain morphological changes in schizophrenia and their relationship to clinical outcome. Biol Psychiatry 31:241–254, 1992

Dever A, Schweizer E: Rapid remission of organic mania after treatment with lorazepam. J Clin Psychopharmacol 8:227, 1988

Dubovsky SL, Thomas M: Psychotic depression: advances in conceptualization and treatment. Hosp Community Psychiatry 43:1189–1198, 1992

Dunner DL: Differential diagnosis of bipolar disorder. J Clin Psychopharmacol 12:75–125, 1992

Dunner DL, Fleiss JL, Fieve RR: Lithium carbonate prophylaxis failure. Br J Psychiatry 129:40, 1976

Escobar JI, Anthony JC, Canino G, et al: Use of neuroleptics, antidepressants, and lithium by U.S. community populations. Psychopharmacol Bull 23:196–200, 1987

Fenton WS, McGlashan TH: National history of schizophrenia subtypes, I: longitudinal study of paranoid, hebephrenic, and undifferentiated schizophrenia. Arch Gen Psychiatry 48:969–977, 1991a

Fenton WS, McGlashan TH: National history of schizophrenia subtypes, II: positive and negative symptoms and long-term course. Arch Gen Psychiatry 48:978–986, 1991b

Frances A, Brown RP, Kocsis JH: Psychotic depression: a separate entity? Am J Psychiatry 138:831–833, 1981

Friedman L, Knutson L, Shurell M, et al: Prefrontal sulcal prominence is inversely related to response to clozapine in schizophrenic patients. Biol Psychiatry 29:865–877, 1991

Friedman L, Lys C, Schulz SC: The relationship of structural brain imaging parameters to antipsychotic treatment response: a review. J Psychiatry Neurosci 17:42–54, 1992

Garfinkel PE, Stancer HC, Persad E: A comparison of haloperidol, lithium carbonate, or either combination in the treatment of mania. J Affect Disord 2:279–288, 1980

Gerner RH: Treatment of acute mania. Psychiatr Clin North Am 16:443–460, 1993

Gerner RH, Post RM, Bunney WE: A dopamine mechanism in mania. Am J Psychiatry 133:1177–1180, 1976

Ghaemi SN, Sachs GS, Baldassano CF, et al: Management of bipolar disorder with adjunctive risperidone: response to open treatment (NR82), in New Research Program and Abstracts: American Psychiatric Association 148th Annual Meeting, Miami, Florida, May 20–25, 1995. Washington, DC, APA, 1995, p 77

Gmur M: A 12-year clinical course of schizophrenia. Soc Psychiatry Psychiatr Epidemiol 26:202–211, 1991

Goodnick PJ: Risperidone treatment of refractory acute mania. J Clin Psychiatry (in press)

Goodwin FK, Jamison KR: Medical treatment of manic episodes, in Manic-Depressive Illness. New York, Oxford University Press, 1990, pp 603–629

Green AI, Alam MY, Sobieraj JT, et al: Clozapine response and plasma catecholamines and their metabolites. Psychiatry Res 46:139–150, 1993

Grossman LS, Harrow M, Goldberg LF, et al: Outcome of schizoaffective disorder at two long-term follow ups. Am J Psychiatry 148:1359–1365, 1991

Harding CM, Zubin J, Strauss JS: Chronicity in schizophrenia: revisited. Br J Psychiatry 161:18:27–37, 1992

Harrow M, Goldberg JF, Grossman LS, et al: Outcome in manic disorders: a naturalistic follow-up study. Arch Gen Psychiatry 47:665–671, 1990

Hasegawa M, Gutierrez-Esteinou R, Way L, et al: Relationship between clinical efficacy and clozapine plasma concentrations in schizophrenia: effect of smoking. J Clin Psychopharmacol 13:383–390, 1993

Helgason L: Twenty years' follow-up of first psychiatric presentation for schizophrenia: what could have been prevented? Acta Psychiatr Scand 81:231–235, 1990

Hillert A, Maier W, Wetzel H, et al: Risperidone in the treatment of disorders with a combined psychotic and depressive syndrome—a functional approach. Pharmocopsychiatr 25:213–217, 1992

Himmelhoch JM, Garfinkel ME: Sources of lithium resistance in mixed mania. Psychopharmacol Bull 22:613–620, 1986

Honigfeld G, Patin J: Predictors of response to clozapine therapy. Psychopharmacology 99(suppl):S64–S67, 1989

Jacobsen FM: Risperidone in the treatment of severe affective illness and refractory OCD (NR275), in New Research Program and Abstracts: American Psychiatric Association 148th Annual Meeting, Miami, Florida, May 20–25, 1995. Washington, DC, APA, 1995, p 129

Janicak PG, Bresnahan DB, Sharma R et al: A comparison of thiothixene and chlorpromazine in the treatment of mania. J Clin Psychopharmacol 8:33–37, 1988

Jimerson DC: Role of dopamine mechanisms in the affective disorders, in Psychopharmacology: The Third Generation of Progress. Edited by Meltzer HY. New York, Raven Press, 1987, pp 505–512

Johnson G, Gershon S, Hekimian LJ: Controlled evaluation of lithium and chlorpromazine in the treatment of manic states: an interim report. Compr Psychiatry 9:563–573, 1968

Johnson G, Gershon S, Burdock EI: Comparative effects of lithium and chlorpromazine in the treatment of acute manic states. Br J Psychiatry 119:267–276, 1971

Johnstone EC, Crow TJ, Frith CD et al: The Northwick Park "functional" psychosis study: diagnosis and treatment response. Lancet 2:119–125, 1988

Juhl RP, Tsuang MT, Perry PJ: Concomitant administration of haloperidol and lithium carbonate in acute mania. Dis Nerv Syst 38:675–676, 1977

Kane J, Honigfeld G, Singer J, et al: Clozapine for the treatment-resistant schizophrenia: a double-blind comparison with chlorpromazine. Arch Gen Psychiatry 45:789–796, 1988

Keck PE Jr, McElroy S-L, Strakowski SM, et al: Pharmacologic treatment of schizoaffective disorder. Psychopharmacology 14:529–538, 1994

Keck PE Jr, Wilson DR, Strakowski SM, et al: Clinical predictors of acute risperidone response in schizophrenia, schizoaffective disorders, and psychotic mood disorders (NR484), in New Research Program and Abstracts: American Psychiatric Association 148th Annual Meeting, Miami, Florida, May 20–25, 1995. Washington, DC, APA, 1995, p 185

Khan A, Cohen S, Stowell M, et al: Treatment options in severe psychotic depression. Convulsive Ther 3:93–99, 1987

Kolakowska T, Wiles DH, McNeilly AS, et al: Correlation between plasma levels of prolactin and chlorpromazine in psychiatric patients. Psychol Med 5:214–216, 1975

Krishna NR, Taylor MA, Abrams RL: Combined haloperidol and lithium carbonate in treating manic patients. Compr Psychiatry 19:119–120, 1978

Krupp P, Barnes P: Leponex-associated granulocytopenia: a review of the situation. Psychopharmacology 99(suppl):S118–S121, 1989

Lamberti JS, Bellnier T, Schwarzkopf SB: Weight gain among schizophrenic patients treated with clozapine. Am J Psychiatry 149:689–690, 1992

Leff J, Sartorius N, Jablensky A, et al: The international pilot study of schizophrenia: five-year follow-up findings. Psychol Med 22:131–145, 1992

Lieberman JA, Sobel SN: Predictors of treatment response and course of schizophrenia. Curr Opinion in Psych 6:63–69, 1993

Lieberman JA, Alvir JMJ, Woerner M, et al: Prospective study of psychobiology in first-episode schizophrenia at Hillside Hospital. Schizophr Bull 18:351–372, 1992a

Lieberman JA, Alvir JMJ, Woerner M, et al: Prospective study of psychobiology in first-episode schizophrenia at Hillside Hospital. Schizophr Bull 19:351–371, 1992b

Loebel AD, Lieberman JA, Alvir JMJ, et al: Duration of psychosis and outcome in first-episode schizophrenia. Am J Psychiatry 149:1183–1188, 1992

Marengo JT, Harrow M, Westermeyer JF: Early longitudinal course of acute-chronic and paranoid undifferentiated schizophrenia subtypes and schizophreniform disorder. J Abnorm Psychol 100:600–603, 1991

Mazure CM, Nelson JC, Jatlow PI, et al: Plasma free homovanillic acid (HVA) as a predictor of clinical response in acute psychosis. Biol Psychiatry 30:475–482, 1991

McElroy SL, Dessain EC, Pope HG, et al: Clozapine in the treatment of psychotic mood disorders, schizoaffective disorder, and schizophrenia. J Clin Psychiatry 52:411–414, 1991

McGlashan T: A selective review of recent North American long-term follow-up studies of schizophrenia. Schizophr Bull 14:515–542, 1988

Meltzer HY: Dopamine and negative symptoms in schizophrenia: critique of the Type I-Type II hypothesis, in Controversies in Schizophrenia: Changes and Constancies. Edited by Alpert M. New York, Guilford, 1985, pp 110–136

Meltzer HY: Clinical studies on the mechanism of action of clozapine: the dopamine-serotonin hypothesis of schizophrenia. Psychopharmacology 99:S18–S27, 1989

Meltzer HY: Dimensions of outcome with clozapine. Br J Psychiatry 160(suppl 17):46–53, 1992a

Meltzer HY: Treatment of the neuroleptic non-responsive schizophrenic patient. Schizophr Bull 18:515–542, 1992b

Meltzer HY: Utilization, multidimensional outcome measures, and risk-benefit considerations for the use of clozapine in schizophrenia, in: Proceedings of the International Academy for Biomedical and Drug Research: New Generation of Antipsychotic Drugs: Novel Mechanisms of Action. International Academy for Biomedical and Drug Research. Milan, Karger Press, 1993, pp 103–117

Meltzer HY: The concept of atypical antipsychotics, in Advances in the Neurobiology of Schizophrenia. Edited by den Boer JA, Westenberg HGM, van Praag HM. England, Wiley (in press)

Meltzer HY, Sommers AA, Luchins DJ: The effect of neuroleptics and other psychotropic drugs on negative symptoms in schizophrenia. J Clin Psychopharmacol 6:329–338, 1986

Meltzer HY, Matsubara S, Lee J-C. Classification of typical and atypical antipsychotic drugs on the basis of dopamine D-1, D-2 and serotonin$_2$ pKi values. J Pharmacol Exp Ther 251:238–246, 1989

Meltzer HY, Okayli G: Reduction of suicidality during clozapine treatment of neuroleptic-resistant schizophrenia: impact on risk benefit assessment. Am J Psychiatry 152:183–190, 1995

Meltzer HY, Yamamoto BK, Lowy MT, et al: The mechanism of action of atypical antipsychotic drugs: an update, in Biology of Schizophrenia and Affective Disease Series, Vol 73. Edited by Watson SJ, Akil H. New York, Raven Press, 1994

Mikuni M, Meltzer HY: Reduction of serotonin-2 receptors in rat cerebral cortex after subchronic administration of imipramine, chlorpromazine, and the combination therapy. Life Sci 34:87–92, 1984

Minter RE, Mandel MR: The treatment of psychotic major depressive disorder with drugs and electroconvulsive therapy. J Nerv Ment Dis 167:726–733, 1979

Moller HJ, Kissling W, Riehl T et al: Double-blind evaluation of the antimanic properties of carbamazepine as a co-medication to haloperidol. Prog Neuropsychopharmacol Biol Psychiatry 13:127–136, 1989

Naber D, Hippius H: The European experience with use of clozapine. Hosp Community Psychiatry 41:886–890, 1990

Naber D, Albus M, Bürke H, et al: Neuroleptic withdrawal in chronic schizophrenia: CT and endocrine variables relating to psychopathology. Psychiatry Res 16:207–219, 1985

Nahunek K, Svestka J, Misurec J, et al: Experiences with clozapine. Cesk Psychiatr 71:11, 1975

Nasrallah HA, Kuperman S, Hamra BJ, et al: Clinical correlates of sulcal widening in chronic schizophrenia. Psychiatry Res 10:237–242, 1983

Nelson JC, Price LH, Jatlow PI: Neuroleptic dose and desipramine concentrations during combined treatment of unipolar delusional depression. Am J Psychiatry 143:1151–1154, 1986

Nimgaonkar VL, Wessely S, Tune LE, et al: Response to drugs in schizophrenia: the influence of family history, obstetric complications and ventricular enlargement. Psychol Med 18:583–592, 1988

Nolen WA: Dopamine and mania. J Affect Disord 5:91–96, 1983

Opler LA, Albert D, Ramirez PM: Psychopharmacologic treatment of negative schizophrenic symptoms. Compr Psychiatry 35:16–28, 1994

Overall JE, Gorham D: The Brief Psychiatric Rating Scale. Psychol Rep 10:149–165, 1962

Parsa M, Ramirez LF, Loula EC, et al: Effect of clozapine on psychotic depression and Parkinsonism. J Clin Psychopharmacol 11:330–331, 1991

Pickar D, Labarca R, Doran AR, et al: Longitudinal measurement of plasma homovanillac acid levels in schizophrenic patients. Arch Gen Psychiatry 43:669–676, 1986

Pickar D, Owen RR, Litman RE, et al: Clinical and biological response to clozapine in patients with schizophrenia. Arch Gen Psychiatry 49:345–353, 1992

Perry PJ, Miller DD, Arndt S, et al: Clozapine concentrations and clinical response in schizophrenic patients. Am J Psychiatry 148:1406–1407, 1991

Post RM: Non-lithium treatment for bipolar disorder. J Clin Psychiatry 51(suppl 8):9–16, 1990

Post RM, Jimerson DC, Bunney WE, et al: Dopamine and mania: behavioral and biochemical effects of the dopamine receptor blocker pimozide. Psychopharmacology 67:297–305, 1980

Post RM, Uhde TW, Roy-Byrne PP et al: Correlates of antimanic response to carbamazepine. Psychiatry Res 21:71–83, 1987

Post RM, Leverich GS, Altahuler L, et al: Lithium discontinuation-induced refractoriness: preliminary observations. Am J Psychiatry 149:1727–1779, 1992

Prien RF, Gelenberg AJ: Alternatives to lithium for preventive treatment of bipolar disorder. Am J Psychiatry 146:840–848, 1989

Prien RF, Coffey EM, Klett AJ: Comparison of lithium carbonate and chlorpromazine in the treatment of mania. Arch Gen Psychiatry 26:146–153, 1972

Rifkin A, Karajgi B, Doddi S, et al: Dose and blood levels of haloperidol in treatment of mania. Psychopharmacol Bull 76:144–146, 1990

Roth BL, Craigo SC, Choudhary MS, et al: Binding of typical and atypical antipsychotic agents to 5-hydroxytryptamine$_6$ (5-HT$_6$) and 5-hydroxytryptamine$_7$(5-HT$_7$) receptors. J Pharmacol Exp Ther 268:1406–1410, 1994

Schmid GB, Stassen HH, Gross G, et al: Long term prognosis of schizophrenia. Psychopathology 24:130–140, 1991

Schnur DB, Mukherjee S, Sackheim HA, et al: Symptomatic predictors of ECT response in medication-nonresponsive manic patients. J Clin Psychiatry 53:63–66, 1992

Schröder J, Geifer FJ, Sauer H: Can computerised tomography be used to predict early treatment response in schizophrenia? Br J Psychiatry 163(suppl 21):13–15, 1993

Scottish Schizophrenia Research Group, MacDonald HL, Best JJK: The Scottish first episode schizophrenia study, VI: computerised tomography brain scans in patients and controls. Br J Psychiatry 154:492–498, 1989

Sernyak MJ, Woods SW: Chronic neuroleptic use in manic-depressive illness. Psychopharmacol Bull 29:375–381, 1993

Shopsin B, Gershon S, Thompson H: Psychoactive drugs in mania. Arch Gen Psychiatry 32:34–42, 1975

Silverstone T, Cookson J: Examining the dopamine hypothesis of schizophrenia and of mania using the prolactin response to antipsychotic drugs. Neuropharmacology 22:539–541, 1983

Singh AN, Catalan J: Risperidone in HIV-related manic psychoses. Lancet 2:1029–1030, 1994

Small JG, Milstein V, Small IF, et al: Computerized EEG structural pathology in schizophrenia: evidence for a selective prefrontal cortical defect. Clin Encephalogr 18:124–135, 1987

Smith RC, Largen J, Calderon M, et al: CT scans and neuropsychological tests as predictors of clinical response in schizophrenics. Psychopharmacol Bull 19:505–509, 1983

Smith RC, Baumgartner R, Ravichandran GK, et al: Cortical atrophy and white matter density in the brains of schizophrenics and clinical response to neuroleptics. Acta Psychiatr Scand 75:11–19, 1987

Spiker DG, Weiss JC, Dealy RS, et al: The pharmacologic treatment of delusional depression. Am J Psychiatry 142:430–436, 1985

Spiker DG, Perel JM, Hanin I, et al: The pharmacologic treatment of delusional depression, part II: J Clin Psychopharmacol 6:339–342, 1986

Suppes T, McElroy SL, Gilbert J, et al: Clozapine in the treatment of dysphoric mania. Biol Psychiatry 32:270–280, 1992

Szymanski S, Lieberman J, Pollack S, et al: Dopamine-serotonin relationship in clozapine response. Psychopharmacology 112 (suppl):S85–S89, 1993

Taylor MA, Abrams R: The phenomenology of mania. A new look at some old patients. Arch Gen Psychiatry 29:520–522, 1973

Taylor MA, Abrams R: Acute mania. Clinical and genetic study of responders and non-responders to treatment. Arch Gen Psychiatry 32:863–865, 1975

Taylor MA, Abrams R: Catatonia. Prevalence and importance in the manic phase of manic-depressive illness. Arch Gen Psychiatry 34:1223–1225, 1977

Taylor MA, Abrams R: Prediction of treatment response in mania. Arch Gen Psychiatry 38:800–803, 1981

Thorup M, Fog R: Clozapine treatment of schizophrenic patients: plasma concentration and coagulation factors. Acta Psychiatr Scand 55:123–126, 1977

Tien AY, Eaton WW: Psychopathologic precursors and sociodemographic risk factors for the schizophrenia syndrome. Arch Gen Psychiatry 49:37–45, 1992

Tohen M, Zarate CA, Centorrino F, et al: Risperidone in the treatment of mania (NR286), in New Research Program and Abstracts: American Psychiatric Association 148th Annual Meeting, Miami, Florida, May 20–25, 1995. Washington, DC, APA, 1995, p 132

Tsoi WF, Wong KE: A 15-year follow-up study of Chinese schizophrenic patients. Acta Psychiatr Scand 84:217–220, 1991

Van Putten T, Marder SR, Wirshing WC, et al: Neuroleptic plasma levels. Schizophr Bull 17:197–216, 1991

Vita A, Sacchetti E, Calzeroni A, et al: Cortical atrophy in schizophrenia: a magnetic resonance imaging study. Psychiatry Res 30:11–20, 1988

Vita A, Dieci M, Giobbio GM, et al: CT scan abnormalities and outcome of chronic schizophrenia. Am J Psychiatry 148:1577–1579, 1991

White E, Cheung P, Silverstone T: Depot antipsychotics in bipolar affective disorder. Int Clin Psychopharmacol 8:119–122, 1993

Winokur G, Coryell W, Akiskal HS et al: Manic-depressive (bipolar) disorders: the course in light of a prospective ten-year follow-up of 131 patients. Acta Psychiatr Scand 89:102–110, 1994

Wyatt RJ: Neuroleptics and the natural course of schizophrenia. Schizophr Bull 17:325–351, 1991

Zelman FP, Hirschowitz J, Garver DL: Mood-incongruent versus mood-congruent psychosis: differential antipsychotic response to lithium therapy. Psychiatry Res 11:317–328, 1985

CHAPTER 8

Electroconvulsive Therapy: Clinical and Biological Aspects

Mitchell S. Nobler, M.D.,
and Harold A. Sackeim, Ph.D.

*I*t has been argued that the study of prediction of response to electroconvulsive therapy (ECT) in major depression is scientifically constrained and of limited clinical significance given the high rate of response to this treatment modality (Abrams 1992; Hamilton 1986); however, there are important reasons for continued research to isolate clinical factors and biological markers that may predict positive outcome. In contrast to early patterns of use, patients now referred for ECT are more diagnostically homogeneous, typically suffering from the most severe depressive illnesses, such as delusional depression and melancholia. Within this more limited diagnostic context, finer distinctions in both clinical and biological parameters must now be made to rationally guide selection of patients who are likely to respond to treatment.

Failure to respond to ECT, given the high expectations associated with this treatment, can lead to demoralization of the patient and his or her family, and may have dire implications for disposition. Further, although initial response rates with ECT are

Preparation of this chapter was supported in part by grants from the National Institute of Mental Health (MH35636 and MH47739) and by a Young Investigator Award from the National Alliance for Research on Schizophrenia and Depression.

impressive, relapse (especially early relapse) after successful course continues to pose problems. Accordingly, we will highlight research on prediction of relapse after ECT. Finally, it should be kept in mind that contemporary ECT patients are often treatment resistant, having failed one or more adequate medication trials. Such medication resistance may have implications for prediction of both initial response to ECT and posttreatment relapse.

Clinical and Demographic Features of Prediction of Response to ECT

Early Studies

Not unlike other somatic treatments in psychiatry, ECT originally was used to treat a variety of patients suffering from a wide range of psychopathology. By the mid 1950s, however, major depressive disorders had become the main clinical indication for ECT. At that time, ECT still predated antidepressant and anxiolytic medications, leaving it as the only somatic treatment for the whole spectrum of mood disorders. Extrapolating from contemporary diagnostic criteria, ECT was likely used to treat syndromes ranging from adjustment disorders, dysthymia, and anxiety-related dysphoria, through severe character pathology and atypical depression, to severe recurrent unipolar and bipolar depression, melancholia, and psychotic depression.

Given such variability in clinical state, there was similar disparity in therapeutic outcome with ECT. Much of the early research in predicting response to ECT was driven by the need to identify particular clinical features and demographic characteristics within the general range of mood disorders. In fact, such ECT outcome prediction studies stimulated considerable interest in the subtyping of depressive disorders, especially the distinction between endogenous/melancholic and reactive/neurotic depression. These early studies have been reviewed in detail before (Abrams 1992; Hamilton 1982); the following is intended as an overview.

Hobson (1953) examined the correlations of 121 clinical characteristics with treatment outcome 2 weeks after ECT. He developed a predictive scale, based on the finding that good response was associated with sudden onset of illness, obvious retardation, good insight, obsessional personality, self-reproach, and a duration of index episode of less than 1 year. Poor response was associated with hypochondriasis, depersonalization, lability, and neurotic and hysterical symptoms. Roberts (1959) assessed 50 female depressed patients 1 month after ECT and found Hobson's scale to be successful in predicting ECT response. Carney and colleagues (1965) assessed outcome at 3 and 6 months after ECT and found favorable response to be predicted by weight loss, early morning awakening, and somatic and paranoid delusions. Unfavorable response was associated with symptoms being worse in the evening, hypochondriasis, anxiety, and hysterical symptoms. Carney and colleagues (1965) noted that all the phenomena that positively correlated with a diagnosis of endogenous depression also had a positive correlation with favorable outcome with ECT. Indeed, this study formed the basis of the Newcastle Scale, used to rate endogenous major depression. Mendels (1967) found similar clinical predictors to those of Hobson and Carney's group; however, the predictive power of these early scales was not universally replicated. For instance, Abrams and colleagues (1973) rated clinical outcome 24 hours after 4–6 ECT treatments (average 4.3) and found no advantage to the above measures, as well as a number of additional clinical and historical features. The relatively early time point of assessment used by these researchers may have clouded a distinction between patients who did and did not respond.

Although some of the early studies were historically important in indicating that certain clinical features (e.g., psychomotor retardation or weight loss) could reliably predict good outcome with ECT, there are important methodological concerns in interpreting their relevance. Foremost is the consideration that the patient populations were probably different from contemporary samples, in part because the diagnostic classification system in use at that time was very different from the present system. There are substantial discrepancies between the DSM-II distinction between psychotic and neurotic depression and the DSM-III distinction between major depression and dysthymia. There is also the question of how clinical response was rated and whether raters were blinded to the putative predictive features. Further, there is the issue of the time of assessment of clinical response, which varied from as little as 24 hours after the fourth ECT to several months after a complete course. Time is particularly critical given the high rates of early relapse with ECT (Sackeim et al. 1990).

A major criticism of early research has been that the predictive rating scales were in essence distilling out patients with severe (perhaps melancholic or delusional) depressions from those with more chronic low-grade (perhaps dysthymic or anxiety-related) or characterological (perhaps atypical) depressive disorders. It is not surprising that the former group of patients would have better outcome with ECT. Indeed, the ability to predict outcome based on symptom features alone may be greatly diminished once patient samples are more diagnostically homogenous. Thus, Pande and colleagues (1988) and Andrade and colleagues (1988) recently found little utility for the older predictive scales within more diagnostically homogeneous samples. Indeed, Andrade and colleagues (1988) concluded that "once an endogenous population is defined, the further application of clinical predictive indices for the selection of patients for ECT is unwarranted" (p. 173).

Diagnosis

Working within the context of patients presenting with major depression, researchers endeavor to isolate individual diagnostic subcategories that are predictive of better outcome; however, it should be remembered that, generally speaking, once a diagnosis of major depression is made, there is a loss of predictive power for one subtype versus another.

Endogenous versus nonendogenous depression.   As reviewed previously, there is ample evidence that ECT is highly effective in endogenous or melancholic depression. Indeed, there is a clinical belief that a diagnosis of melancholia, by itself, predicts good ECT outcome. But, do patients with melancholia fare better with ECT than nonmelancholic depressives? The answer may be no. Coryell and Zimmerman (1984) unexpectedly found that patients with melancholia tended to have poorer global clinical ratings at discharge than nonmelancholic patients, and had significantly more symptoms at follow-up. This group later replicated the finding that the presence of melancholia in a depressed sample had little relation to ECT outcome (Zimmerman et al. 1985). A related belief is that specific endogenous symptoms in any given patient (whether or not he or she meets criteria for endogenous or melancholic depression) are more likely to remit with ECT than nonendogenous symptoms. In fact, the only study in this area found no support for this concept. Drawing from a larger sample, Prudic and colleagues (1989) identified 20 patients who met Research Diagnostic Criteria (Spitzer et al. 1978) for endogenous depression and who had a partial response to ECT (blind clinical evaluation immediately after a completed ECT course). Using symptom scores on the Hamilton Rating Scale for Depression (Hamilton 1960), three different subscales were formulated to characterize endogenous features. Prudic's group found no evidence that endogenous symptoms were more responsive to ECT than nonendogenous symptoms. A third related issue is whether any specific symptom feature in melancholic patients is predictive of good ECT response. Again, the findings have been negative, as Abrams and Vedak (1991) found no individual Hamilton Depression Rating Scale (HDRS) item that could predict outcome after six ECT treatments in a sample of 47 male patients with melancholic depression.

Delusional depression (psychotic depression). Perhaps even stronger than the belief in the utility of ECT for severe melancholia is the view that ECT is a particularly effective treatment for depressions with associated psychotic features. Stated differently, most clinicians believe that the presence of delusions among patients with major depression predicts good response to ECT. Overall, there is strong empirical support for this contention. Indeed, in the large British trials of real versus simulated ECT (anesthesia alone), a consistent predictor of response to real ECT was the presence of delusions (Buchan et al. 1992; Clinical Research Centre 1984). In a retrospective study, Dunn and Quinlan (1978) also found the presence of delusions to predict good ECT response. Further, in a sample of medication-resistant patients, Mandel and colleagues (1977) found the presence of delusions to predict positive outcome. Others have also found that the presence of delusions predicts better outcome at discharge (Coryell and Zimmerman 1984; Pande et al. 1990); however, Rich and colleagues (1986) found that psychotic and nonpsychotic depressed patients showed equal benefit from ECT. It is worth noting that patients in this study were allowed to remain on concurrent medications, including neuroleptics, and that nonpsychotic patients had significantly shorter duration of the index episode. One early study found that the absence of paranoid symptoms was related to better response to ECT (Hamilton and White 1960). On the whole, however, most studies find that the presence of psychotic symptoms is predictive of good outcome with ECT, or at least makes no measurable difference. The interpretation of this empirical observation remains open. At face value, it may be that psychotic depression is uniquely responsive to ECT, and at a rate that exceeds that in nonpsychotic depression. An alternative explanation derives from the finding that patients with demonstrated medication resistance (which will be discussed later in this chapter) are less likely to respond to ECT than patients without such treatment resistance (Prudic et al. 1990). Particularly since antidepressant pharmacotherapy alone is not sufficient treatment for delusional depression (Spiker et al. 1985), many patients with this illness are referred for ECT without ever being proven as medication resistant. It would be predicted that such patients would fare better with ECT than nonpsychotic patients who had failed to respond to adequate medication trials.

Double depression.   There are no studies that document the percentage of patients referred for ECT who are suffering from a major depressive episode superimposed on chronic dysthymia (double depression). Based on evidence that patients with double depression respond as well to antidepressant medications as patients with major depressive disorder alone, Prudic and colleagues (1993) compared the effects of ECT on 75 patients with major depressive disorder and 25 patients with double depression. Of note, the patients with double depression were an average of 10 years younger than patients with major depressive disorder. Prudic and colleagues (1993) found that patients with double depression (especially those with more severe symptoms at baseline) were just as likely to respond to ECT as patients with major depressive disorder, but that patients with double depression who responded had more residual depressive symptoms than patients with major depressive disorder who responded both immediately and 1 week after a completed course of ECT. These findings suggest that patients with double depression are as likely to achieve remission with ECT from their major depressive episode as patients with major depressive disorder alone, but that some residual symptoms in patients with double depression after ECT may represent a return to a dysthymic baseline.

Duration of Illness

In his classic study, Hobson (1953) indicated that a shorter duration of the index episode of depression (1-year cutoff) was a predictor of good ECT response. This finding was subsequently confirmed by several other groups (Coryell and Zimmerman 1984; Dunn and Quinlan 1978; Fraser and Glass 1980; Hamilton and White 1960; Kindler et al. 1991), although some studies found no relation or a weaker relation between duration of index episode and clinical outcome (Andrade et al. 1988; Mendels 1967; Sackeim et al. 1987a). If anything, then, a shorter index episode of depression may be associated with an increased likelihood of favorable ECT response.

Severity of Illness

Roberts (1959) originally reported that higher symptom scores at baseline predicted better ECT response. In contrast, Andrade and colleagues (1988) and Sackeim and colleagues (1987a) found no differences in initial severity between patients who did and did not respond. At the other extreme, some investigators have reported that patients who did not respond to ECT had greater initial severity of depression (Kindler et al. 1991; Pande et al. 1988). Thus, there is no consensus on how symptom severity, independent of the presence of psychosis or melancholia, is predictive of ECT response.

Patient Age

An association between increased age and favorable response to ECT has been reported by several authors (Carney et al. 1965; Coryell and Zimmerman 1984; Mendels 1967; Nystrom 1964; Roberts 1959; Sackeim et al. 1987a). Others have reported that age has no relation to outcome (Andrade et al. 1988; Hamilton and White 1960; Hobson 1953). In contrast, Ottosson (1960) and Rich and colleagues (1984) found increasing age to be associated with a lower rate of ECT response. On the whole, there is a statistical effect for older age (measured as a continuous variable) to be predictive of better ECT response, but this effect is of doubtful clinical significance.

Treatment History

There is increasing awareness of patients who suffer from depression and are resistant to treatment with conventional antidepressant medications (Roose and Glassman 1990). In fact, the lack of response to antidepressant pharmacotherapy is now perhaps the most common indication for ECT. This represents a significant change from the prepharmacological era in which ECT was a first-line treatment for depression. This shift in referral patterns should not be underestimated as a factor in predicting ECT outcome. Moreover, most studies of both clinical and biological predictors fail to control for medication resistance.

Medication resistance. As ECT becomes more of a second- and third-line treatment for depression, there is reason to believe that response rates will be affected. For instance, it had been previously suggested that ECT outcome was poorer for medication-resistant patients compared with non–medication-resistant patients (Hamilton 1974; Medical Research Council 1965). More recently, Prudic and colleagues (1990) rated 53 patients as to the adequacy of pre-ECT medication trials in the index episode. Among 24 patients rated as medication resistant, there was only a 50% response rate to bilateral ECT as opposed to an 86% response rate among patients who were not known to be medication resistant. These findings argue against the long-held clinical impression that ECT has consistently good outcome, regardless of medication treatment history. Although response rates on the order of 50% are still impressive, especially among patients with established resistance to other somatic treatments, the presence of medication resistance may predict poorer outcome with ECT relative to its absence. Furthermore, medication resistance may underlie the associations of poor ECT outcome with episode duration and the presence of delusions. In terms of the former, patients with the longest depressive episodes often receive lengthier and more numerous medication trials before ECT, and are more likely to qualify as medication resistant (Prudic et al. 1990). In contrast, patients with psychotic depression often receive inadequate pharmacologic treatment (i.e., they do not receive combination antipsychotic-antidepressant medication) or are referred for ECT either earlier in their episode, or as a first-line treatment.

Psychotherapy. There are no reports of the impact of psychotherapy during a depressive episode on the success or failure of ECT later in the same episode. In other words, it is unknown whether failure to respond to an adequate course of psychotherapy predicts good or poor response to ECT. With the growing popularity of short-term techniques such as interpersonal psychotherapy, such research will become more relevant, and hopefully more feasible.

Prediction of Response to ECT: Biological Factors

Early Research

There were a few early attempts to develop biological tests that would predict outcome with ECT. These are reviewed in detail elsewhere (Hamilton 1982). One interesting example of this type of work was the sedation threshold test, developed by Roth and colleagues (1957) and Shagass and colleagues (1956; Shagass 1957). The test essentially involved an assessment of the dose of intravenous barbiturate necessary to cause sedation (e.g., nystagmus, slurred speech, or electroencephalographic changes). The Shagass group (1956) found that low threshold (less requirement for barbiturate) predicted better clinical improvement with ECT; however, this same sedation threshold range also differentiated "psychotic" from "neurotic" depression. In other words, this physiological test appeared to distinguish more severe from less severe depressions (and possibly depression from schizophrenia), thus accounting for its ability to predict treatment outcome. Though potentially useful as a diagnostic marker, the sedation threshold test lacked reliability and was ultimately abandoned (see Hamilton 1982).

Anesthetic Sensitivity

A recent study reexamined the potential utility of anesthetic threshold in forecasting ECT response (Barry et al. 1991). The authors monitored sensitivity to methohexital anesthesia (loss of eyelash reflex) throughout a course of ECT. While anesthetic sensitivity changed in many patients over the course of ECT, the direction of change had no relation to immediate clinical outcome. In contrast, change in methohexital threshold did predict relapse (methohexital threshold as a predictor of treatment outcome is discussed later in this chapter).

Neuroendocrine Challenge Tests

Dexamethasone suppression test (DST).   Of all the possible biological predictors of ECT outcome, the DST has received the most research attention and has been the subject of several critical reviews (Coryell 1986; Kamil and Joffe 1991; Ribeiro et al. 1993; Scott 1989). There continues to be some uncertainty about the utility of the DST in forecasting ECT outcome. Studies have examined the relation of baseline DST status to clinical outcome, the prognostic significance of converting abnormal to normal (or vice versa) over a course of ECT, and the relation of posttreatment DST status to relapse (also discussed later in this chapter).

Coryell (1982) reported that an abnormal baseline DST predicted good ECT outcome by global clinical rating, but not by HDRS scores. Other researchers were not able to replicate this finding (Devanand et al. 1987, 1991; Katona and Aldridge 1984; Katona et al. 1987; Lipman et al. 1986a). Similarly, early reports that normalization of the DST during a course of ECT predicts recovery (e.g., Albala et al. 1981) were not replicated (Lipman et al. 1986b) and conflict with evidence that many patients who respond to ECT in fact convert from a normal to an abnormal DST status (Devanand et al. 1987, 1991). Finally, a recent study emphasized the need for measuring plasma dexamethasone levels concurrent with cortisol assays (Devanand et al. 1991). These authors found that patients who responded to ECT had larger progressive increases in plasma dexamethasone levels than patients who did not respond to ECT, but that these changes were more evident one week post-ECT than immediately after the ECT course.

Thyrotropin-releasing hormone (TRH) stimulation test. There have been a few reports on the thyroid-stimulating hormone (TSH) response to TRH in patients treated with ECT. One group of researchers has reported increases in TSH response to TRH after a course of ECT and subsequently used these values to predict relapse (Krog-Meyer et al. 1984). In contrast, Decina and colleagues (1987) found that the TSH response became more blunted after ECT and also had no value in predicting outcome. A recent report confirmed that the TRH stimulation test is of dubious value in predicting ECT response (Lyskouras et al. 1993).

Neurophysins

Neurophysins are carrier peptides for the posterior pituitary hormones oxytocin and vasopressin. The oxytocin-associated neurophysin is referred to as hNpII, which can be assayed from blood. Scott and colleagues (1989, 1991) reported that the acute surge in hNpII immediately after the first ECT treatment predicted clinical improvement after the completed course of treatment. The same group recently demonstrated that the amount of oxytocin released after an ECT-induced seizure is greater with higher intensity simulation (Riddle et al. 1993). The authors speculate that the relation of the oxytocin (and consequently, hNpII) surge and clinical response is mediated by effects of stimulus intensity. Indeed, there is evidence that the degree to which stimulus intensity exceeds patients' seizure thresholds (see below) is a strong determinant of ECT response, at least for unilateral ECT (Sackeim et al. 1987a, 1993).

The work with oxytocin and hNpII was not without methodological flaws, such as controlling for concurrent psychotropic medications and conducting separate analyses for response to bilateral and unilateral ECT. Yet, although these data require independent replication, they hold promise as isolating a predictor of initial ECT response. They also highlight the possibility that biological changes sensitive to stimulus intensity may be greater at initial ECT treatments relative to those later in the course of treatment.

Biopterin Metabolism

Abnormalities in biopterin metabolism have been reported in depression (Coppen et al. 1989). Tetrahydrobiopterin (BH_4) is a cofactor crucial to the biosynthetic pathways of the biogenic amines. The relative ratio of neopterins to biopterins (N:B) in the urine is an index of the synthesis of BH_4, with an elevated ratio implying a failure to produce BH_4. Anderson and coworkers (1992) measured the urinary N:B ratio in 23 depressed patients before and after a course of ECT and in 26 normal control subjects. At baseline, depressed patients had a higher N:B ratio than the control subjects. Upon further analysis, patients who went on to respond to ECT had higher ratios than control subjects, whereas nonresponders did not differ from control subjects.

Seizure Physiology

Seizure threshold.   Seizure threshold can be defined as the minimum electrical stimulus intensity necessary to elicit a generalized seizure of adequate duration (i.e., 20–25 seconds). Using a stimulus titration procedure, the Columbia University group has provided evidence that there is a wide range in seizure threshold among patients, and that electrical stimulus dose relative to seizure threshold is a more critical determinant of therapeutic efficacy with ECT than the absolute electrical dose administered (Sackeim et al. 1987a, 1993). In a study comparing the efficacy of bilateral and right unilateral ECT, given at stimulus doses just above the seizure threshold, it was found that greater increase in seizure threshold over a course of ECT was significantly associated with greater symptom reduction (Sackeim et al. 1987b). In the same study, no increase or minimal increase in seizure threshold during the ECT course predicted poor clinical response. Others have also reported that the absence of a significant rise in seizure threshold during a course of ECT is associated with poor outcome (Roemer et al. 1990; Yatham et al. 1989).

Cerebral blood flow.   Cerebral blood flow increases dramatically during induced or spontaneous seizures, then falls below resting levels in the postictal period. As part of the research protocol at Columbia, depressed patients referred for ECT were assessed using the planar 133-xenon inhalation technique in order to measure cortical cerebral blood flow. Fifty-four patients were studied just before and 50 minutes after the sixth ECT treatment. It was found that patients who went on to respond to ECT had significantly greater decreases in both global and regional cortical cerebral blood flow than patients who did not respond (Nobler et al. 1993a). To determine whether these effects were sufficiently consistent to be useful in prediction of ECT outcome, a predictive discriminant function analysis was performed (unpublished data). Overall classification accuracy was strong (likelihood ratio $\chi^2 = 16.18, P < .0001$). Of the 28 patients who responded to ECT, 19 (68%) were correctly classified. Of note, 22 of 26 (85%) patients who did not respond to ECT were correctly classified. This aspect was particularly critical, since presumably the greatest clinical need pertains to the identification of patients who will not respond. The logistic regression associated with this classification analysis indicated that topographic alterations in cerebral blood flow acutely following ECT may be particularly important in forecasting clinical outcome. It should be noted that the data set pertained to changes in cerebral blood flow primarily at the sixth ECT treatment. As there may have already been cumulative changes in cerebral blood flow during the first part of the ECT course, the data may have underestimated effect sizes and classification accuracy.

Recent electroencephalographic studies.   There is evidence that generalized seizures of adequate duration can reliably be elicited in ECT that are weak in therapeutic properties (Sackeim et al. 1987a, 1993). Attention has been recently focused on features of the seizure other than duration that might be predictive of good response. For example, right unilateral ECT given at a stimulus intensity just above seizure threshold (i.e., a low, weakly therapeutic dose) produced seizures that differed in a number of respects on electroencephalograms (EEGs) from seizures produced by higher dosage unilateral ECT or bilateral ECT. These included a longer time to make a transition from polyspike to slow-wave activity and less bioelectric suppression immediately after seizure termination (Nobler et al. 1993b). Bilateral ECT given at stimulus intensities well above seizure threshold (strongly therapeutic) resulted in seizures with the greatest EEG slow-wave amplitude (Nobler et al. 1993b). Others have reported similar findings (Krystal et al. 1993). The implication of this work is that potential ictal

EEG markers can be identified that predict good or poor ECT response. Indeed, one manufacturer of ECT devices has added indices purported to measure the quality of the ictal EEG. As yet, there has been no testing of the sensitivity or specificity of these measures in predicting ECT outcome.

> *Case 1: Response prediction.*   The patient was a 71-year-old man with a long history of bipolar affective disorder. His first depressive episode occurred at the age of 22, for which he received ECT. Up until 1965, the patient received 10 more courses of ECT. He was later placed on lithium, and remained well until 1988, when the lithium had to be discontinued because of secondary renal insufficiency. He then suffered an episode of psychotic depression and recovered on valproate and perphenazine. He subsequently became depressed again, but could not tolerate nortriptyline. He was admitted for ECT on a regimen of 24 mg of perphenazine and 100 mg of trazodone. He entered our study protocol and received 10 bilateral ECT treatments at a dosage just above his seizure threshold, which was unusually high. The patient did not respond, but then received nine treatments at a dose approximately 100% above seizure threshold, which was achieved by using extreme settings on a custom-modified ECT device (Sackeim et al. 1987a). The patient responded to these further treatments and was discharged after being prescribed carbamazepine. He subsequently relapsed and received a course of bilateral ECT at another institution. He was noted to have a poor response to this conventional ECT regimen.

This case illustrates several practical issues regarding the prediction of a given individual's response to ECT. He had difficulty achieving adequate doses of antidepressant medications, which is not uncommon among elderly patients. Therefore, by contemporary standards, he was not medication resistant. Taken together with his advanced age, a history of ECT response, and the presence of psychotic features, one might have predicted good response to ECT. This expectation was ultimately met, but only with the high-dosage treatment that could be provided by a special ECT device. The importance of such technical factors as dosage relative to seizure threshold was later reinforced in this case by the poor response to conventional ECT at lower stimulus intensity.

Prediction of Relapse After Successful ECT

Clinical Factors

Diagnosis. There has been no systematic study of the impact of diagnostic subtype on relapse after ECT. In a study comparing patients with double depression with patients with major depressive disorder alone (Prudic et al. 1993), there was a trend for greater 1-year relapse rates among patients with double depression (75%) as opposed to major depressive disorder (54%); however, the small sample size limited confidence in this finding.

Medication resistance Sackeim and colleagues (1990) conducted a prospective naturalistic study of relapse rates in 58 patients who were followed up to 1 year after ECT. The patients were rated for their degree of medication resistance in the index episode before ECT using a method similar to that of Prudic and colleagues (1990). In the majority of cases, continuation pharmacotherapy was at the discretion of the patient's private physician. Relapse after ECT was twice as common in patients who were medication resistant before ECT than in nonresistant patients. Furthermore, among medication-resistant patients, the adequacy of continuing pharmacotherapy had no impact on relapse rates. This finding calls into question the practice of prescribing the same medication after ECT that failed to elicit a response before ECT. Indeed, for the medication-resistant patient who does respond to ECT, careful thought should be given to alternative psychopharmacologic strategies as well as the possibility of continuing ECT.

Biological Factors

Insulin resistance. Based on reports of both abnormal glucose metabolism in depression and of ECT effects on glucose metabolism, Williams and colleagues (1992) monitored plasma insulin and glucose during a course of ECT in 20 patients. Both insulin and glucose peaked immediately after ECT administration. The greatest insulin peak occurred after the first ECT. The nine patients who relapsed at 2 months had significantly lower insulin peaks at the fifth ECT relative to patients who remained euthymic.

Anesthetic sensitivity. In the study by Barry and colleagues (1991), 52% of the patients relapsed 12 months after ECT. The authors reported that patients who relapsed demonstrated an increased anesthetic sensitivity during the ECT course (i.e., they had a decreased requirement for methohexital).

Neurophysins. Scott and colleagues (1989) initially reported that baseline serum hNpII was lower in patients with sustained clinical improvement 2 months after ECT. This finding was not replicated in their subsequent expanded sample (Scott et al. 1991). In contrast to their finding that maximum hNpII release after the first ECT predicted initial clinical improvement, they found no significant relation between maximal hNpII release and clinical outcome at 2 months (Scott et al. 1991).

Neuroendocrine challenge tests. The examination of whether the DST can predict relapse has not yielded promising results, with the majority of studies finding the test to be of limited use (Coryell 1986; Devanand et al. 1991; Ribeiro et al. 1993). Indeed, studies have reported results that were the opposite of initial expectations. For example, Coryell and Zimmerman (1983) reported that patients whose DST normalized over the course of ECT had a poorer outcome at 6 months than patients who experience no change in DST results. Lipman and colleagues (1986b) had similar findings. Furthermore, Katona and colleagues (1987) found the DST to be unsuccessful at predicting 6-month outcome. As mentioned, it has been suggested that ECT will have the relatively acute effect of corrupting DST results in many patients (Coryell 1986; Devanand et al. 1991). This raises the issue of choosing an appropriate time for administering the DST after ECT. Again, in line with the findings of Devanand and colleagues (1991) that post-DST dexamethasone levels were altered by ECT, there has been no study of the value of the DST in predicting relapse that has taken post-DST dexamethasone levels into account.

Krog-Meyer and colleagues (1984) reported that patients with greater TSH response to TRH after ECT relative to pretreatment baseline were the least likely to relapse. Decina and colleagues (1987) were unable to replicate these findings.

Case 2: Relapse prediction.   The patient was a 63-year-old woman with a history of bipolar affective disorder with onset in her mid 40s. In the summer of 1991, she suffered an episode of major depression and responded to a course of ECT at another institution. She quickly relapsed, and was treated with 300 mg of carbamazepine and 1 mg of haloperidol per day, followed by nortriptyline (with adequate blood levels). She was felt to be improved by September 1991; however, she relapsed again, and experienced no improvement during inadequate trials of trazodone and bupropion. The patient received eight right unilateral ECT treatments with poor response. She then responded to crossover treatment with seven bilateral, high-dosage treatments. She was discharged on sertraline and lorazepam, but relapsed again in 2 months. She later went on to receive continuation ECT at another institution.

This case illustrates the difficulty in predicting who will relapse after successful treatment with ECT. Although this patient was not resistant to medications in the index episode (she did not receive adequate pharmacotherapy), she nonetheless suffered early relapse. Thus, although medication resistance may be predictive of relapse, clearly the absence of such treatment resistance does not guarantee a lack of relapse. Other factors must then be entertained to account for relapse in patients such as this.

Conclusion

It appears that there are several logical steps that the clinician can take in order to identify patients who will respond to ECT. As with any treatment selection process in medicine, a careful diagnostic assessment should be the starting point. For the psychiatric patient, before ECT is recommended, the presence of a major depressive episode should be verified. Though preliminary, a diagnosis of double depression should not be cause for pessimism; however, an extremely long current episode of major depression may decrease the chance of good ECT response. Other factors, such as symptom severity and patient age, in and of themselves, probably have less impact on eventual outcome.

After such thorough clinical assessment, consideration should be given to the adequacy of pharmacological treatment in the index episode. The initial evidence suggests that a proven history of medication resistance, particularly in relation to tricyclic antidepressants, may decrease the chance of favorable ECT outcome. Given the ever-expanding pharmacotherapeutic armamentarium, this factor may become increasingly important in predicting ECT outcome; however, even here, many patients with medication resistance will demonstrate strong short-term response.

As patient samples treated with ECT have become more diagnostically homogeneous, research has turned to biological tests to identify potential ECT responders. Early enthusiasm for neuroendocrine challenge tests has abated as further studies have cast doubt on their predictive accuracy. A novel approach using a pretreatment measure to predict outcome is the assay of urinary biopterins. This work requires replication. Other new approaches exploit the dynamic physiological responses to the ECT-induced seizure, as opposed to baseline measures. Examples are release of neurophysins and insulin after seizures, changes in seizure threshold, the degree of change in cerebral blood flow with ECT, and features of the ictal EEG. Such "on-line" assessment of treatment adequacy, with associated objective biological markers, offers the distinct advantage of allowing the clinician to alter ECT administration (e.g., adjust stimulus dose relative to seizure threshold) early in the course of treatment.

In predicting which patients are more likely to relapse after ECT, most findings remain preliminary. This is often a secondary concern of ECT research. Yet, for the larger public health issues of morbidity and rehospitalization, this is no less critical a topic. At present, a clinical history of resistance to antidepressant medications is perhaps the best predictor of relapse after recovery with ECT.

References

Abrams R: Electroconvulsive Therapy. New York, Oxford University Press, 1992

Abrams R, Vedak C: Prediction of ECT response in melancholia. Convulsive Ther 7:81–84, 1991

Abrams R, Fink M, Feldstein S: Prediction of clinical response to ECT. Br J Psychiatry 122:457–460, 1973

Albala AA, Greden JF, Tarika J, et al: Changes in serial dexamethasone suppression tests among unipolar depressive receiving electroconvulsive treatment. Biol Psychiatry 16:551–560, 1981

Anderson DN, Abou-Saleh MT, Collins J, et al: Pterin metabolism in depression: an extension of the amine hypothesis and possible marker of response to ECT. Psychol Med 22:863–869, 1992

Andrade C, Gangadhar BN, Swaminath G, et al: Predicting the outcome of endogenous depression following electroconvulsive therapy. Convulsive Ther 4:169–174, 1988

Barry S, Rowan MJ, Mulhall J, et al: Change in barbiturate anaesthetic sensitivity as a prognostic indicator of electroconvulsive therapy outcome. Acta Psychiatr Scand 83:251–255, 1991

Buchan H, Johnstone E, McPherson K, et al: Who benefits from electroconvulsive therapy? Combined results of the Leicester and Northwick Park trials. Br J Psychiatry 160:355–359, 1992.

Carney MWP, Roth M, Garside RF: The diagnosis of depressive syndromes and the prediction of ECT response. Br J Psychiatry 111:659–674, 1965

Clinical Research Centre: Division of Psychiatry: The Northwick Park ECT trial: predictors of response to real and simulated ECT. Br J Psychiatry 144:227–237, 1984

Coppen A, Swade C, Jones SA, et al: Depression and tetrahydrobiopterin: the folate connection. J Affect Disord 16:103–107, 1989

Coryell W: Hypothalamic-pituitary-adrenal axis abnormality and ECT response. Psychiatry Res 6:283–291, 1982

Coryell W: Are serial dexamethasone suppression tests useful in electroconvulsive therapy? J Affect Disord 10:59–66, 1986

Coryell W, Zimmerman M: The dexamethasone suppression test and ECT outcome: a six-month follow-up. Biol Psychiatry 18:21–27, 1983

Coryell W, Zimmerman M: Outcome following ECT for primary unipolar depression: a test of newly proposed response predictors. Am J Psychiatry 141:862–867, 1984

Decina P, Sackeim HA, Kahn DA, et al: Effects of ECT on the TRH stimulation test. Psychoneuroendocrinology 12:29–34, 1987

Devanand DP, Decina P, Sackeim HA, et al: Serial dexamethasone suppression tests in initial suppressors and nonsuppressors treated with electroconvulsive therapy. Biol Psychiatry 22:463–472, 1987

Devanand DP, Sackeim HA, Lo ES, et al: Serial dexamethasone suppression tests and plasma dexamethasone levels: effects of clinical response to electroconvulsive therapy in major depression. Arch Gen Psychiatry 48:525–533, 1991

Dunn CG, Quinlan D: Indicators of ECT response and non-response in the treatment of depression. J Clin Psychiatry 39:620–622, 1978

Fraser RM, Glass IB: Unilateral and bilateral ECT in elderly patients. A comparative study. Acta Psychiatr Scand 62:13–31, 1980

Hamilton M: A rating scale for depression. J Neurol Neurosurg Psychiatry 23:56–62, 1960

Hamilton M: Drug resistant depressions: response to ECT. Pharmacopsychiatry 7:205–206, 1974

Hamilton M: Prediction of the response of depressions to ECT, in Electroconvulsive Therapy: Biological Foundations and Clinical Applications. Edited by Abrams A, Essman WB. New York, Spectrum Publications, 1982, pp 113–127

Hamilton M: Electroconvulsive therapy. Indications and contraindications. Ann NY Acad Sci 462:5–11, 1986

Hamilton M, White J: Factors related to the outcome of depression treated with ECT. J Ment Sci 106:1031–1041, 1960

Hobson RF: Prognostic factors in ECT. J Neurol Neurosurg Psychiatry 16:275–281, 1953

Kamil R, Joffe RT: Neuroendocrine testing in electroconvulsive therapy. Psychiatr Clin North Am 14:961–970, 1991

Katona CL, Aldridge CR: Prediction of ECT response. Neuropharmacology 23:281–283, 1984

Katona CL, Aldridge CR, Roth M, et al: The dexamethasone suppression test and prediction of outcome in patients receiving ECT. Br J Psychiatry 150:315–318, 1987

Kindler S, Shapira B, Hadjez J, et al: Factors influencing response to bilateral electroconvulsive therapy in major depression. Convulsive Ther 7:245–254, 1991

Krog-Meyer I, Kirkegaard C, Kijne B, et al: Prediction of relapse with the TRH test and prophylactic amitriptyline in 39 patients with endogenous depression. Am J Psychiatry 141:945–948, 1984

Krystal AD, Weiner RD, McCall WV, et al: The effects of ECT stimulus dose and electrode placement on the ictal electroencephalogram: an intraindividual crossover study. Biol Psychiatry 34:759–767, 1993

Lipman RS, Backup C, Bobrin Y, et al: Dexamethasone suppression test as a predictor of response to electroconvulsive therapy, I: inpatient treatment. Convulsive Ther 2:151–160, 1986a

Lipman RS, Uffner W, Schwalb N, et al: Dexamethasone suppression test as a predictor of response to electroconvulsive therapy, II: six-month follow-up. Convulsive Ther 2:161–167, 1986b

Lyskouras L, Markianos M, Augoustides A, et al: Evaluation of TSH and prolactin responses to TRH as predictors of the therapeutic effect of ECT in depression. Eur Neuropsychopharmacol 3:81–83, 1993

Mandel MR, Welch CA, Mieske M, et al: Prediction of response to ECT in tricyclic-intolerant or tricyclic-resistant depressed patients. McLean Hosp J 2:203–209, 1977

Medical Research Council: Clinical trial of the treatment of depressive illness. BMJ 5439:881–886, 1965

Mendels J: The prediction of response to electroconvulsive therapy. Am J Psychiatry 124:153–159, 1967

Nobler MS, Sackeim HA, Solomou M, et al: EEG manifestations during ECT: Effects of electrode placement and stimulus intensity. Biol Psychiatry 34:321–330, 1993a

Nobler MS, Sackeim HA, Prohovnik I, et al: Effects of ECT on regional cerebral blood flow in mood disorders. Biol Psychiatry 33:65A–66A, 1993b

Nystrom S: On relation between clinical factors and efficacy of ECT in depression. Acta Psychiatr Neurol Scand 181(suppl):11–135, 1964

Ottosson J: Experimental studies of the mode of action of electroconvulsive therapy. Acta Psychiatr Scand 145(suppl):1–141, 1960

Pande AC, Krugler T, Haskett RF, et al: Predictors of response to electroconvulsive therapy in major depressive disorder. Biol Psychiatry 24:91–93, 1988

Pande AC, Grunhaus LJ, Haskett RF, et al: Electroconvulsive therapy in delusional and non-delusional depressive disorder. J Affect Disord 19:215–219, 1990

Prudic J, Devanand DP, Sackeim HA, et al: Relative response of endogenous and non-endogenous symptoms to electroconvulsive therapy. J Affect Disord 16:59–64, 1989

Prudic J, Sackeim HA, Devanand DP: Medication resistance and clinical response to electroconvulsive therapy. Psychiatry Res 31:287–296, 1990

Prudic J, Sackeim HA, Devanand DP, et al: The efficacy of ECT in double depression. Depression 1:38–44, 1993

Ribeiro SCM, Tandon R, Grunhaus L, et al: The DST as a predictor of outcome in depression: a meta-analysis. Am J Psychiatry 150:1618–1629, 1993

Rich CL, Spiker DG, Jewell SW, et al: The efficiency of ECT; I: Response rate in depressive episodes. Psychiatry Res 11:167–176, 1984

Rich CL, Spiker DG, Jewell SW, et al: ECT response in psychotic versus nonpsychotic unipolar depressives. J Clin Psychiatry 47:123–125, 1986

Riddle WJR, Scott AIF, Bennie J, et al: Current intensity and oxytocin release after electroconvulsive therapy. Biol Psychiatry 33:839–841, 1993

Roberts JM: Prognostic factors in the electroshock treatment of depressive states: (1) clinical features from history and examination. J Ment Sci 105:693–702, 1959

Roemer RA, Dubin WR, Jaffe R, et al: An efficacy study of single- versus double-seizure induction with ECT in major depression. J Clin Psychiatry 51:473–478, 1990

Roose SP, Glassman AH: Treatment Strategies for Refractory Depression. Washington, DC, American Psychiatric Press, 1990

Roth M, Kay DW, Shaw J, et al: Prognosis and pentothal induced electro-encephalographic changes in electro-convulsive treatment: an approach to the problem of regulation of convulsive therapy. Electroencephalogr Clin Neurophysiol 9:225–237, 1957

Sackeim HA, Decina P, Kanzler M, et al: Effects of electrode placement on the efficacy of titrated, low-dose ECT. Am J Psychiatry 144:1449–1455, 1987a

Sackeim HA, Decina P, Portnoy S, et al: Studies of dosage, seizure threshold, and seizure duration in ECT. Biol Psychiatry 22:249–268, 1987b

Sackeim HA, Prudic J, Devanand DP, et al: The impact of medication resistance and continuation pharmacotherapy on relapse following response to electroconvulsive therapy in major depression. J Clin Psychopharmacol 10:96–104, 1990

Sackeim HA, Prudic J, Devanand DP, et al: Effects of stimulus intensity and electrode placement on the efficacy and cognitive effects of electroconvulsive therapy. N Engl J Med 328:839–846, 1993

Scott AI: Which depressed patients will respond to electroconvulsive therapy? The search for biological predictors of recovery. Br J Psychiatry 154:8–17, 1989

Scott AI, Whalley LJ, Legros JJ: Treatment outcome, seizure duration, and the neurophysin response to ECT. Biol Psychiatry 25:585–597, 1989

Scott AI, Shering PA, Legros JJ, et al: Improvement in depressive illness is not associated with altered release of neurophysins over a course of ECT. Psychiatry Res 36:65–73, 1991

Shagass C: A measurable neurophysiological factor of psychiatric significance. Electroencephalogr Clin Neurophysiol 9:101–108, 1957

Shagass C, Naiman J, Mihalik J: An objective test which differentiates between neurotic and psychotic depression. Arch Neurol Psychiatry 75:461–471, 1956

Spiker DG, Weiss JC, Dealy RS, et al: The pharmacological treatment of delusional depression. Am J Psychiatry 142:430–438, 1985

Spitzer RL, Endicott J, Robins E: Research diagnostic criteria: rationale and reliability. Arch Gen Psychiatry 35:773–782, 1978

Williams K, Smith J, Glue P, et al: The effects of electroconvulsive therapy on plasma insulin and glucose in depression. Br J Psychiatry 161:94–98, 1992

Yatham LN, Barry S, Dinan TG, et al: Which patients will respond to ECT? Br J Psychiatry 154:879–80, 1989

Zimmerman M, Coryell W, Pfohl B: The treatment validity of DSM-III melancholic subtyping. Psychiatry Res 16:37–43, 1985

CHAPTER 9

Comment and Review

David L. Dunner, M.D.

*T*he purpose of this chapter is to summarize the discussion of predictors of treatment response in patients with mood disorders. The development of predictor response is an interesting topic because knowledge regarding the characteristics that are related to response to particular treatments would simplify the clinical management of patients with mood disorders and would also help develop hypotheses regarding the etiology of mood disorders. Numerous investigators over the past few decades have attempted to define the biology of mood disorders in order to understand how these illnesses evolve and therefore predict treatment; however, there is no proven test that is well correlated with treatment response. In fact, there is more abundant data on patients with mood disorders who respond to placebo than on predictors of treatment outcome.

This chapter reviews the previous contributions to further the understanding of predictors of response, including the related diagnostic aspects (symptoms in particular), psychological aspects, familial factors, and biological factors. Also considered is the response to a variety of treatments, including psychotherapies and pharmacotherapies.

Diagnostic Issues

To clarify treatment response, it is important to determine the diagnosis of subjects being studied and to have a sample group that is as homogeneous as possible. Over the past 100 years, there have been several attempts to separate mood disorders into meaningful subcategories. In the 1960s, the separation of depression into bipolar (having a history of mania) and unipolar (absence of mania) disorders seemed to be quite useful. This separation was clinically based on histories of patients with mood disorders and was initially supported by clinical factors and family history data (Angst 1966; Leonhard et al. 1962; Perris 1966). Further refinement of the bipolar-unipolar classification resulted in the separation of patients into those with depression and hypomania (bipolar II), those with severe mania (bipolar I), and those with depression only (unipolar) (Dunner et al. 1976b).

The delineation of bipolar II as a separate subtype had certain advantages. First, it strengthened the homogeneity of the bipolar I subtype. Indeed, most studies of patients who are hospitalized for mania show bipolar I patients to be more similar in terms of clinical, familial, outcome, and treatment characteristics than other subtypes (Dunner 1983, 1993; Fieve and Dunner 1975). Bipolar II patients also seem to be relatively homogeneous and fairly stable over their course of illness (Dunner 1993; Dunner et al. 1976a). Second, the separation of bipolar II patients from those who might have been called unipolar has helped to provide a clearer definition of true unipolar disorder. It should be noted, however, that unipolar depression (or major depression, as classified in DSM-III-R) describes an extremely heterogeneous population probably characterized by a number of etiologies, courses of illness, biological factors, and clinical characteristics.

Interestingly, when looking at family characteristics of affective disorders, the strongest genetic loading for depression appears to be among relatives of bipolar I and bipolar II patients; this is in contrast to unipolar patients, in whom only a small increase in depression was found over the population frequency (Coryell et al. 1985; Fieve et al. 1984; Gershon et al. 1982). Therefore, clinicians interested in a disorder with high genetic loading (and presumably a biological correlation) should start with studies of patients who have bipolar disorders; these patients are more likely to reveal biological factors and prediction of treatment outcome than those with unipolar disorders.

Given that bipolar I, bipolar II, and unipolar patients may differ, some treatment outcome studies suggest differential results.

For example, in one study testing the catecholamine hypothesis of mood disorders, L-dopa was administered to depressed patients. The response noted during the L-dopa administration was interesting because unipolar depressed patients showed no response; bipolar II depressed patients had an antidepressant response; and bipolar I depressed patients had manic or psychotic-like responses (Gershon et al. 1971). This appears to be the only study showing a differential treatment outcome for bipolar I, bipolar II, and unipolar depressed patients. Other studies suggested that the antidepressant response of patients with bipolar I depression to tricyclic antidepressants (TCAs) was poor compared with their response to monoamine oxidase inhibitors (MAOIs), particularly tranylcypromine (Himmelhoch et al. 1989; Thase et al. 1992). This was discussed in greater detail in Chapters 1 and 2. In addition, hypomania may be seen in bipolar (I or II) depressed patients who are treated with a variety of antidepressant medications, although it is unusual that treatment-emergent hypomania would occur in unipolar patients. An antidepressant response to the administration of lithium was noted in bipolar (I and II) patients but not in unipolar patients (Goodwin et al. 1972). In a very small study, the administration of L-tryptophane, used to test the hypothesis of a serotonin deficit in depression, resulted in an antidepressant response in a few bipolar I and bipolar II patients but not in unipolar patients (Farkas et al. 1976).

Rapid cycling has been reported to occur when tricyclic medications are administered to bipolar depressed patients (Wehr and Goodwin 1979). The response to treatment with newer nontricyclic antidepressants tends to be quite similar among bipolar I, bipolar II, and unipolar depressives; however, as discussed in Chapter 3, some preliminary results have shown that bupropion may be particularly useful in bipolar depression.

Regarding depression symptoms, there is perhaps more correlation of symptoms with treatment response among individual unipolar patients than antidepressant response among unipolar patients as a group. For example, there is a large body of literature that describes patients who have "atypical depression" and who are characterized by anxiety, hypochondriasis, reversed neurovegetative symptoms (oversleeping and overeating), feeling worse in the evening than in the morning, rejection sensitivity, mood reactivity, and a feeling of leaden paralysis. Studies supporting a differential treatment response in such patients have shown better response to MAOIs (particularly phenelzine) and bupropion (Goodnick and Extein 1989; Liebowitz et al. 1988; Quitkin et al. 1991; Stewart et al. 1993; West and Dally 1959). Chapters 1–3 provided further elaboration on the critique of studies regarding TCAs, MAOIs, and selective serotonin reuptake inhibitors (SSRIs), respectively.

Patients with severe depression characterized by melancholia have seemed to respond poorly to psychotherapy and better to medication or electroconvulsive therapy (ECT) (Avery et al. 1983; Bielski and Friedel 1976; Charney and Nelson 1981; Stewart et al. 1993). Depressed patients with psychotic symptoms responded more favorably to ECT and (to a lesser extent) a combination of an antidepressant and antipsychotic treatment than to an antidepressant or antipsychotic medication alone (Avery et al. 1983; Crow and Johnstone 1986; Khan et al. 1993; Prudic et al. 1990). This was discussed in greater detail in Chapter 8.

Depressed patients who are described as having a seasonal pattern responded better to light therapy than other depressed patients (Bauer and Dunner 1993; Rosenthal et al. 1984; Terman et al. 1989).

In terms of response to TCAs, the literature supports the notion that psychomotor-retarded patients responded less well to the more sedating tertiary amine TCAs than to the secondary amine TCAs; in contrast, patients with anxiety and sleeplessness preferentially responded to treatment with the more sedating tertiary amine TCAs (Avery et al. 1983; Bielski and Friedel 1976; Nelson and Charney 1981). These results led to the notion that TCAs were either activating or sedating, which is probably a misconception, because TCAs tend to be sedating whether they are tertiary or secondary amines (the issue is the degree of sedation). Most patients with hypersomnia and psychomotor retardation did not tolerate treatment with the more sedating TCAs. For the most part, TCAs are given at bedtime whether they are "activating" or "sedating," and this fact belies the notion of these general categories. Unfortunately, this characterization has extended into the era of the SSRIs. In general, SSRIs are neither sedating nor activating; because they are not especially sedating, however, they have been characterized as activating. There was a clinical supposition that the SSRIs would not be effective in patients whose depression was characterized by anxiety; however, reviewing the SSRIs as a group has tended to show response in a broad spectrum of patients with a variety of symptoms, including those with anxiety accompanying their depression (Beasley et al. 1991; Dunbar et al. 1991; Feighner 1985; Schatzberg et al. 1987; Stokes 1993). Evidence concerning psychomotor retardation as a predictor of response to fluoxetine or agitation as a predictor of response to fluvoxamine was further discussed in Chapter 3. Bupropion, one of the newer drugs, is considered an activating compound. In the author's experience, it has worked best in patients with psychomotor retardation and somewhat less well in patients with anxiety, panic, or sleep disturbance. Recent data have suggested that panic attacks accompanying depression may be associated with higher suicide and suicide attempt rates than depression uncomplicated by these anxiety features (Coryell et al. 1982; Weissman et al. 1989). One of the difficulties with SSRIs is an induction of anxiety in some patients. For this reason, if using an SSRI, it may be beneficial to start with lower than recommended doses in the treatment of depressed patients with panic attacks, although the treatment outcome in such patients is usually satisfactory. The presence of associated syndromes of obsessive-compulsive disorder , panic, and posttraumatic stress disorder with depression as a predictor of response to SSRIs was discussed in Chapter 3.

Patients whose depression has lasted 2 years or more may not respond to treatment as well as patients who have more acute depressive episodes. Indeed, in characterizing depressed patients who respond to placebo, one feature that has seemed to hold true across a number of studies is that the patients most likely to respond to placebo treatment tend to be those with acute onsets of rather severe depression or recurrent depressive histories. Patients less likely to respond to placebo treatment were those whose depression was of longer duration (Khan et al. 1989, 1991). Thus, chronic depression may be more difficult to treat than acute onset depression.

Factors predicting response to maintenance therapy are not well delineated. Bipolar patients with a rapid-cycling course respond less well to lithium and to other mood stabilizers than do patients who have a regular course of bipolar disorder (Bauer and Whybrow 1993; Dunner and Fieve 1974; Dunner et al. 1977). This parameter was examined in greater detail in Chapters 4–6, which discuss lithium and anticonvulsants.

In summary, diagnostic and symptom issues seem to have some impact on treatment choice; however, in the individual patient, there is no easily defined symptom cluster that necessarily leads to the use of a particular treatment. For example, some depressed anergic patients respond to sedating TCAs, whereas some anxious depressed patients respond to bupropion or the less-sedating TCAs. Thus, choosing a drug that may not seem appropriate for the patient's symptoms may sometimes have beneficial effects.

Psychological Aspects

In terms of the discussion of chronic depression above, it has been found that patients with treatment-resistant depression who have failed to respond to multiple treatment trials tend to have personality characteristic alterations as measured by the Tri-Dimensional Personality Questionnaire (Cloninger 1987; Nelsen and Dunner 1993; Nelsen and Dunner 1995). Such patients have less novelty-seeking behavior and more harm-avoidance behavior than non–treatment-resistant depressed patients. This implies that chronicity of depression and treatment resistance (since they are related) may result in personality changes, causing these patients to be less likely to respond to treatment.

The issue of Axis II disorders (or personality disorders) is certainly a complicated one because most of these disorders do not show high rates of diagnostic interrupter reliability; thus, their diagnosis may be considered suspect (Docherty et al. 1986; Frances and Widiger 1986). Indeed, it is often useful to consider the longitudinal interpersonal characteristics of a patient before ascertaining a personality disorder diagnosis, rather than how the patient appears cross-sectionally during a depressed phase. An example is someone who has the flu and is irritable and cranky. This individual's personality appears to be negative and irritable, reflecting the state of the illness rather than a trait characteristic. Personality should be reviewed as a trait or long-standing characteristic; it should not necessarily be regarded as something that could be affected by the occurrence of depression, but that which endures the depression's remission.

There are some depressed patients who warrant the diagnosis of a personality disorder. Unfortunately, when a patient meets the criteria for one personality disorder, it is likely that criteria will also be met for several other personality disorders, raising doubt as to what is being described as a personality disorder. It is clear, however, that the presence of personality disorders has a negative impact on treatment outcome (Flick et al. 1993; Reich and Green 1991; Shea et al. 1990). There is a paucity of data on this possible predictor of response to SSRIs; however, Chapter 1 offered what is known regarding personality disorders as a predictor of response to TCAs.

Severity of depression seems to have some bearing on treatment response. A review of data from the National Institute of Mental Health depression treatment trial suggests that patients with more severe depression responded better to treatment with imipramine than to treatment with the interpersonal and cognitive psychotherapies studied. Patients with less severe depression tended to have a high number of side effects, subsequently dropping out of the imipramine treatment study. Thus, these psychotherapies may be preferable for the mildly depressed patient (Elkin et al. 1989).

Whether or not some patients could respond to a particular form of psychotherapy based on their personality makeup is not clear. Cognitive and interpersonal psychotherapies, therefore, are different in their approach to the patient, but it is not known if patients would show a preferential response to one or the other.

Family History Predictors of Response

There is a clinical lore that patients with family members who have responded to a particular medication for treatment of a depressive illness are perhaps likely to themselves respond to the same medication. What confounds this view is that when a patient gets better during treatment, it does not necessarily mean that the treatment itself caused the improvement. Depressive illness has a natural history, and most patients with depression improve whether treated or not. Thus, controlled data are sparse that would permit the assessment of a patient's family history of treatment response as a predictor of treatment response in that patient. Clinical and anecdotal experience must be relied upon instead (Pare 1962). As a general clinical guideline, if a family member has responded to treatment with a particular medication, it is certainly worthwhile to try that medication with the depressed patient. It must be realized, however, that because individuals share genes with relatives only to a certain extent, genetic makeups of individuals (except for identical twins) are distinctive. If there are genetic factors that mitigate response, these may differ within and between families. Assortative mating has also been shown to occur with a certain degree of regularity in patients with mood disorders (Colombo et al. 1990; Gershon et al. 1973). This suggests that a patient's relative who is depressed may have a different genetic etiology of depression than the patient.

There has been a suggestion that maintenance response to lithium in bipolar patients is correlated with a positive family history of mania (Mendlewicz et al. 1973); further elaboration of this was found in Chapter 4. Other results appear to challenge this idea, however. First, patients experiencing rapid cycling usually do not benefit from lithium trials, either early on or as maintenance treatment. The family histories of patients who experience rapid cycling showed the same degree of risk for mania as the family histories of bipolar patients who do not experience rapid cycling, suggesting that family history of mania does not predict lithium maintenance outcome (Dunner et al. 1977; Nurnberger et al. 1988). Furthermore, lithium maintenance outcome is likely to change. Patients who have done well on lithium for a certain period of time may have their first affective episode after several years of long-term treatment; thus, lithium may not be effective in some patients indefinitely (Fleiss et al. 1978). Second, family history can change if a relative develops a manic disorder (i.e., a negative family history changes to positive). Both of these factors, therefore, can change in a such a direction that would negate the conclusion that family history is associated with lithium maintenance response. Yet, it is curious that with regard to anticonvulsants, a negative family history is a useful predictor for response to carbamazepine, whereas a positive family history is a predictor for response to valproate (see Chapters 5 and 6).

Some studies have suggested that there may be at least two types of unipolar depression: depressive spectrum disease (depressed women who have family histories of alcoholism and depression) and pure depressive disease (depressed men with late onset of depression who have family histories of depression only) (Winokur et al. 1971, 1978). Unfortunately, these unipolar depressive subtypes have not been supported by treatment outcome studies in showing a differential response to pharmacotherapy.

In summary, family history is not a good indication for treatment.

Biological Predictors of Response

Factors associated with severe depression or melancholia correlate with a lack of placebo response. Thus, short REM latencies and positive dexamethasone suppression tests (DSTs) are two factors that may be more positive in melancholic patients or severely depressed patients; however, the correlation of short REM latency or positive DST result with a particular antidepressant is not well documented (Ribeiro et al. 1993; Rush et al. 1985, 1989); it may be interesting to note, however, that a negative DST result has been associated with response to MAOIs. Additional details on these factors was provided in Chapters 1–3.

There has been a suggestion that levels of norepinephrine metabolites correlate with treatment outcome. This was based on the theory that related low levels of norepinephrine to depression, the so-called catecholamine hypothesis of mood disorders (Bunney and Davis 1965; Schildkraut 1965). This hypothesis led to the study of norepinephrine metabolites, in particular 3-methoxy-4-hydroxy-phenylglycol (MHPG). It was stated that low levels of MHPG may predict response, especially to treatment with secondary amine TCAs (predominantly noradrengeric), and that high levels of MHPG may predict response to amitriptyline (or other antidepressants that are predominantly serotonergic) (Beckmann and Goodwin 1975; Maas et al. 1972; Schatzberg et al. 1983). The dexedrine or methylphenidate stimulation test also theoretically predicted outcome to response. This test was further discussed in Chapter 1. Patients who were given stimulants and who showed a response within 24 hours were supposedly better responders to noradrengeric-type TCAs than to serotonergic TCAs. In general, these findings tended to correlate with the clinical description of patients, with low levels of MHPG found in depressed patients with psychomotor retardation and higher levels found in depressed patients with agitation and sleeplessness. It is interesting to note that these correlations have not proven to be exact, and the use of MHPG as a predictor is no longer given overall credence. Further discussion regarding specific cases in which MHPG might yet have some usefulness can be found in Chapters 1 and 3.

Other attempts to look at biological factors as predictors include studies of a serotonin metabolite, 5-hydroxyindoleactic acid (5-HIAA). One report found that low levels of 5-HIAA in cerebrospinal fluid (CSF) correlated with suicidal behavior among depressed patients (Brown and Goodwin 1986; Van Praag 1984); however, there are only a few studies that show CSF 5-HIAA as a predictor of treatment response. Other serotonin parameters include the ration of tryptophan to neutral amino acid, platelet serotonin levels, and neuroendocrine challenge tests. These future potential predictors are discussed in Chapters 1 and 3.

Because most patients respond to the use of any antidepressant within 4–6 weeks of treatment, predictors may not have a crucial role in all treatment cases. This comes as a consequence of the overlap of biochemical effects of currently available antidepressants; for example, amitriptyline and fluoxetine affect both norepinephrine and serotonin levels, although to different degrees. Furthermore, it is known that many interactions exist between biochemical systems. Although an agent may be serotonin specific, that effect on serotonin may produce secondary changes in both dopamine and norepinephrine.

Conclusion

It is important to remember that when assessing treatment outcome, just because a patient responds during treatment does not necessarily mean the treatment was associated with the response. In the past, attempts to predict treatment outcome have been based largely on hypotheses concerning the etiology of mood disorders. Methodological problems in these studies included failure to define the population in a homogeneous way and difficulty in ascertaining the response itself. It is hoped that future studies of the biology of mood disorders will help uncover better prediction of treatment response.

References

Angst J: Zur Ätiologie und Nosologie endogener depressiver Psychosen. Berlin, Springer Verlag, 1966

Avery DH, Wilson LG, Dunner DL: Diagnostic subtypes of depression as predictors of therapeutic response, in Treatment of Depression: Old Controversies and New Approaches. Edited by Clayton PJ, Barrett JE. New York, Raven Press, 1983, pp 193–204

Bauer MS, Dunner DL: Validity of seasonal pattern as a modifier for recurrent mood disorders for DSM-IV. Compr Psychiatry 34:159–170, 1993

Bauer M, Whybrow P: Validity of rapid cycling as a modifier for bipolar disorder in DSM-IV. Depression 1:11–19, 1993

Beasley CM Jr, Sayler ME, Bosomworth JC, et al: High dose fluoxetine: efficacy and activating-sedating effects in agitated and retarded depression. J Clin Psychopharmacol 11:166–174, 1991

Beckmann H, Goodwin FK: Antidepressant response to tricyclics and urinary MHPG in unipolar patients. Arch Gen Psychiatry 32:17–21, 1975

Bielski RJ, Friedel RO: Prediction of antidepressant response. Arch Gen Psychiatry 33:1479–1489, 1976

Brown GL, Goodwin FK: Cerebrospinal fluid correlates of suicide attempts and aggression. Ann NY Acad Sci 487:175–188, 1986

Bunney WE Jr, Davis J: Norepinephrine in depressive reactions. Arch Gen Psychiatry 13:483–494, 1965

Charney DS, Nelson JC: Delusional and non-delusional unipolar depression: further evidence for distinct subtypes. Am J Psychiatry 138: 328–333, 1981

Cloninger CR: A systematic method for clinical description of personality variants. Arch Gen Psychiatry 44:573–588, 1987

Colombo J, Cox G, Dunner DL: Assortative mating in affective and anxiety disorders: preliminary findings. Psychiatric Genetics 1:35–44, 1990

Coryell W, Noyes R, Clancy J: Excess mortality in panic disorder. Arch Gen Psychiatry 39:701–703, 1982

Coryell W, Endicott J, Andreason N, et al: Bipolar I, bipolar II, and non-bipolar major depression among the relatives of affectively ill probands. Am J Psychiatry 142: 817–821, 1985

Crow TJ, Johnstone EC: Controlled trials of electroconvulsive therapy. Ann NY Acad Sci 462:12–29, 1986

Docherty JP, Fiester SJ, Shea T: Syndrome diagnosis and personality disorder, in Psychiatry Update: American Psychiatric Association Annual Review, Vol 5. Edited by Frances AJ, Hales RE. Washington, DC, American Psychiatric Press, 1986, pp 315–355

Dunbar GC, Cohn JB, Fabre LF, et al: A comparison of paroxetine, imipramine and placebo in depressed outpatients. Br J Psychiatry 159:394–398, 1991

Dunner DL: Subtypes of bipolar affective disorder with particular regard to bipolar II. Psychiatr Dev 1:75–86, 1983

Dunner DL: A review of the diagnostic status of "Bipolar II" for the DSM-IV work group on mood disorder. Depression 1:2–10, 1993

Dunner DL, Fieve RR: Clinical factors in lithium carbonate prophylaxis failure. Arch Gen Psychiatry 30:229–233, 1974

Dunner DL, Fleiss JF, Fieve RR: The course of development of mania in patients with recurrent depression. Am J Psychiatry 133:905–908, 1976a

Dunner DL, Gershon ES, Goodwin FK: Heritable factors in the severity of affective illness. Biol Psychiatry 11:31–42, 1976b

Dunner DL, Patrick V, Fieve RR: Rapid cycling manic depressive patients. Compr Psychiatry 18:561–566, 1977

Elkin I, Shea MT, Watkins JT, et al: National Institute of Mental Health Treatment of Depression Collaborative Research Program: general effectiveness of treatments. Arch Gen Psychiatry 46:971–982, 1989

Farkas T, Dunner DL, Fieve RR: L-Tryptophan in depression. Biol Psychiatry 11:295–302, 1976

Feighner JP: A comparative trial of fluoxetine and amitriptyline with major depressive disorder. J Clin Psychiatry 45:369–373, 1985

Fieve RR, Dunner DL: Unipolar and bipolar affective states, in The Nature and Treatment of Depression. Edited by Flach FF, Draghisc SC. New York, Wiley, 1975, pp 145–166

Fieve RR, Go R, Dunner DL, et al: Search for biological/genetic markers in a long-term epidemiological and morbid risk study of affective disorders. J Psychiatr Res 18:425–445, 1984

Fleiss JL, Prien RF, Dunner DL, et al: Actuarial studies of the course of manic-depressive illness. Compr Psychiatry 19:335–362, 1978

Flick SM, Roy-Byrne PP, Cowley DS, et al: DSM-III-R personality disorders in a mood and anxiety disorders clinic: prevalence, comorbidity, and clinical correlates. J Affect Disord 27: 71–79, 1993

Frances AJ, Widiger T: The classification of personality disorders: An overview of problems and solutions, in Psychiatry Update: American Psychiatric Association Annual Review, Vol 5. Edited by Frances AJ, Hales RE. Washington, DC, American Psychiatric Press, 1986, pp 240–257

Gershon ES, Bunney WE Jr, Goodwin FK, et al: Catecholamines and affective illness: studies with L-dopa and alpha-methyl-para-tyrosine, in Brain Chemistry and Mental Disease. Edited by Ho BT, McIssac WM. New York, Plenum Press, 1971, pp 135–161

Gershon ES, Dunner DL, Stuart L, et al: Associative mating in the affective disorders. Biol Psychiatry 7:63–74, 1973

Gershon ES, Hamovit J, Guroff JJ, et al: A family study of schizoaffective, bipolar I, bipolar II, unipolar and normal control probands. Arch Gen Psychiatry 39:1157–1167, 1982

Goodnick PJ, Extein IL: Bupropion and fluoxetine in depressive subtypes. Ann Clin Psychiatry 1:119–122, 1989

Goodwin FK, Murphy DL, Dunner DL, et al: Lithium response in unipolar versus bipolar depression. Am J Psychiatry 129:44–47, 1972

Himmelhoch JM, Thase ME, Mallinger AG, et al: Tranylcypromine versus imipramine in anergic bipolar depression. Am J Psychiatry 148:910–916, 1989

Khan A, Cohen S, Dager S, et al: Onset of response in relation to outcome in depressed outpatients with placebo and imipramine. J Affect Disord 17:33–38, 1989

Khan A, Dager SR, Avery DH, et al: Chronicity of depressive episode in relation to antidepressant-placebo response. Neuropsychopharmacology 4:125–130, 1991

Khan A, Mirolo H, Hughes D, Bierut L: Electroconvulsive therapy. Psychiatr Clin North Am 16:497–513, 1993

Leonhard K, Korff I, Schultz H: Die Temperamente in den Familien der monopolaren and bipolaren phasischen Psychosen. Psychiatr Neurol 143:416–434, 1962

Liebowitz MR, Quitkin FM, Stewart JW, et al: Antidepressant specificity in atypical depression. Arch Gen Psychiatry 45:129–138, 1988

Maas JW, Fawcett JA, Dekirmenjian H. Catecholamine metabolism, depressive illness, and drug response. Arch Gen Psychiatry 26:252–262, 1972

Mendlewicz J, Fieve RR, Stallone F: Relationship between effectiveness of lithium therapy and family history. Am J Psychiatry 130:1011–1013, 1973

Nelsen MR, Dunner DL: Treatment resistance in unipolar depression and other disorders: diagnostic concerns and treatment possibilities. Psychiatr Clin North Am 16:541–566, 1993

Nelsen M, Dunner DL: Clinical and differential diagnostic aspects of treatment resistant depression. J Psychiatr Res 29:43–50, 1995

Nelson JC, Charney DJ. The symptoms of major depressive illness. Am J Psychiatry 138:1–13, 1981

Nurnberger JI Jr., Guroff JJ, Hamovit J, et al: A family study of rapid-cycling bipolar illness. J Affect Disord 15:87–91, 1988

Pare CMB: Differentiation of two genetically specific types of depression by the response to antidepressants. Lancet 2:1340–1343, 1962

Perris C: A study of bipolar (manic-depressive) and unipolar recurrent depressive psychoses. Acta Psychiatr Scand 42(suppl 194):1–188, 1966

Prudic J, Sackheim HA, Devanand DP: Medication resistance and clinical response to electroconvulsive therapy. Psychiatry Res 31:287–296, 1990

Quitkin FM, Harrigan W, Stewart JW, et al: Response to phenelzine and imipramine in placebo nonresponders with atypical depression: a new application of the crossover design. Arch Gen Psychiatry 48:319–323, 1991

Reich JH, Green AI: Effect of personality disorders on outcome of treatment. J Nerv Ment Dis 179:74–82, 1991

Ribeiro SCM, Tandon R, Grunhaus L, et al: The DST as a predictor of outcome in depression: a meta-analysis. Am J Psychiatry 150:1618–1629, 1993

Rosenthal NE, Sach DA, Gillin JC, et al: Seasonal affective disorder: a description of the syndrome and preliminary findings with light therapy. Arch Gen Psychiatry 41:72–80, 1984

Rush AJ, Erman MK, Schlesser MA, et al: Alprazolam versus amitriptyline in depressions with reduced REM latencies. Arch Gen Psychiatry 42:1154–1159, 1985

Rush AJ, Giles DE, Jarrett RB, et al: Reduced REM latency predicts response to tricyclic medication in depressed outpatients. Biol Psychiatry 26:61–72, 1989

Schatzberg AF, Orsulak PJ, Rosenbaum AH, et al: Biochemical subtypes of unipolar depressives, in Treatment of Depression: Old Controversies and New Approaches. Edited by Clayton PJ, Barrett JE. New York, Raven Press, 1983, pp 53–60

Schatzberg A, Dessain E, O'Neill P, et al: Recent studies on selective serotonergic antidepressants: trazodone, fluoxetine, and fluvoxamine. J Clin Psychopharmacol 7:44–49, 1987

Schildkraut JJ: The catecholamine hypothesis of affective disorder: a review of supporting evidence. Am J Psychiatry 122:509–522, 1965

Shea MT, Pilkonis PA, Beckham E, et al: Personality disorders and treatment outcome in the NIMH treatment of depression collaborative research program. Am J Psychiatry 147:711–718, 1990

Stewart JW, McGrath PJ, Rabkin JG, et al: Atypical depression: a valid clinical entity? Psychiatr Clin North Am 16:479–495, 1993

Stokes PE: Fluoxetine: a five-year review. Clin Ther 15:216–243, 1993

Terman M, Terman JS, Quitkin F, et al: Light therapy for seasonal affective disorder: a review of efficacy. Neuropsychopharmacology 2:1–22, 1989

Thase ME, Mallinger AG, McKnight BS, Himmelhoch JM: Treatment of imipramine-resistant recurrent depression, IV: a double-blind crossover study of tranylcypromine for anergic bipolar depression. Am J Psychiatry 149:195–198, 1992

Van Praag HM: Depression, suicide, and serotonin metabolism in the brain, in Neurobiology of Mood Disorders. Edited by Post RM, Ballenger JC. Baltimore, MD, Williams & Wilkins, 1984, pp 601–618

Wehr TA, Goodwin FK: Rapid cycling in manic-depressives induced by tricyclic antidepressants. Arch Gen Psychiatry 36:552–559, 1979

Weissman MM, Klerman GL, Markowitz JS, et al: Suicide ideation and suicide attempts in panic disorder and attacks. N Engl J Med 321:1209–1214, 1989

West ED, Dally PJ: Effect of iproniazid in depressive syndromes. BMJ 1:1491–1494, 1959

Winokur G, Cadoret R, Dorzab J, et al: Depressive disease: a genetic study. Arch Gen Psychiatry 24:135–144, 1971

Winokur G, Behar D, Vanvalkenburg C, et al: Is a familial definition of depression both feasible and valid? J Nerv Ment Dis 166:764–768, 1978

Index

*Page numbers printed in **boldface** type refer to tables or figures.*